Celestial Healing

of related interest

Vital Healing
Energy, Mind and Spirit in Traditional Medicines of India, Tibet
and the Middle East—Middle Asia
Marc S. Micozzi, MD, PhD
with Donald McCown, MAMS, MSS and Mones Abu-Asab, PhD
(Unani), Hakima Amri, PhD (Unani), Kevin Ergil, MA, MS, LAc
(Tibet), Howard Hall, PsyD, PhD (Sufi), Hari Sharma, MD (Maharishi
Ayurveda, Introduction, Conclusion, and Appendix), Kenneth G. Zysk,
DPhil, PhD (Ayurveda and Siddha)
ISBN 978 1 84819 045 0

Wan's Clinical Application of Chinese Medicine
Scientific Practice of Diagnosis, Treatment and Therapeutic
Monitoring
Giorgio Repeti, LAc, with Marc S. Micozzi, MD, PhD
ISBN 978 1 84819 047 4

Ayurvedic Healing
Contemporary Maharishi Ayurvedic Medicine and Science
Hari Sharma, MD, DABP, FCAP, FRCPC, DABHM and
Christopher Clark, MD
Medical Editor: Marc S. Micozzi, MD, PhD
ISBN 978 1 84819 069 6

Chinese Medical Qigong
Editor in Chief: Tianjun Liu, OMD
Associate Editor in Chief: Kevin W. Chen, PhD
Foreword by Marc S. Micozzi, MD, PhD
ISBN 978 1 84819 023 8

Celestial Healing

Energy, Mind and Spirit in Traditional Medicines
of China, and East and Southeast Asia

Marc S. Micozzi, MD, PhD

*with Kevin Ergil, MA, MS, LAc (Chinese
Medicine and Acupuncture, Qi, and Qi Gong),
Laurel S. Gabler, BA, MSc (Thai Medicine),
and Kerry Palanjian, MBA (Shiatsu)*

SINGING
DRAGON

LONDON AND PHILADELPHIA

First published in 2011
by Singing Dragon
an imprint of Jessica Kingsley Publishers
116 Pentonville Road
London N1 9JB, UK
and
400 Market Street, Suite 400
Philadelphia, PA 19106, USA

www.singingdragon.com

Library of Congress Cataloging in Publication Data
A CIP catalog record for this book is available from the Library of Congress

British Library Cataloguing in Publication Data
A CIP catalogue record for this book is available from the British Library

ISBN 978 1 84819 060 3

Printed and bound in the United States

Contents

Part I: China

Part II: East Asia

Part III: Southeast Asia

Part IV: Chinese Medicine in the West and Worldwide

Acknowledgments

I would like to acknowledge the following colleagues for their insights, perspectives, and scholarship on the medicines of China and Asia: Alicia Micozzi, EMT, WMT; Amy Ai, PhD; David Mayor, MA, BAc, MBAcC; Donald Bisson, RRPr; Donald McCown, MAMS, MSS, LSW; Efrem Korngold, OMD; Gerard Bodeker, EdD; Giorgio Repeti, LAc; Harriet Beinfield, OMD; Judith DeLany, LMT; Kerry Palanjian, MBA; Kevin Ergil, MA, MS, LAc; Marnae Ergil, MA, MS, LAc; Stanley Burns, MD; and Terry Oleson, PhD.

Special thanks to The Henry Luce Foundation, New York, NY, for awarding me a Luce Scholarship, and to The Asia Foundation, San Francisco, CA, for providing support in the field, for my original research in East and Southeast Asia.

Chronological Phases of Chinese Medicine

⚘

Dynasty	Dates	Philosophy	Medical Practice	Classic Texts
Shang	1770– 1120 BC	Magico- religious	Shamanism; ancestors	*Oracle bones*
Zhou	1120– 220 BC	Magico- religious; Confucius; Lao Zi	Shamanism; Demons; herbalism	
Qin	220– 206 BC		Acupuncture; Moxibustion; Qi gong	*Divine Husbandman's Materia Medica*; *Yellow Emperor's Classic of Internal Medicine*
Han	206 BC– 220 AD			
Daoist Rebellion and Interregnum	221–265			*Nan Jing Classic of Difficult Issues*
Jin	266–420			
Sixteen Kingdoms	421–580			

Dynasty	Dates	Period	Developments	Texts
Sui and Tang	581–959			*Classic of Spells*
Sung	960–1279		Formal medical education; Medical specialization	
Yuan	1280–1367		Advances in acupuncture; Herbalism	*Treatise on Cold Diseases*
Ming	1368–1644	Naturalistic	Peak of acupuncture and moxibustion	*Discourses on Warm Diseases, Acupuncture Great Compendia*
Qing (Manchu)	1644–1911		Acupuncture declines	
Republic*	1912–1936	"Modern"	Western medicine	
Manchukuo	1937–1945	Japanese occupation		
People's Republic	1949–	Communism	"Traditional Chinese medicine"	*Barefoot Doctors' Manual*

*Republic of China (1912) continues on island of Taiwan, formerly Formosa

Preface

Chinese medical knowledge and practice manifests a number of forms mixed with a broad range of *ethnomedical* traditions found in the region of "Greater China" throughout East and Southeast Asia. The historic influence of a "Greater China," concomitant with the advance and expansion of Chinese civilization through the centuries, extends east to Korea and Japan and south to Indochina, the Malay Peninsula, and the Indonesian Archipelago. In addition to the spread of Chinese cultural, political, and economic influence throughout these areas, there were also millions of "overseas Chinese" who migrated to these regions and maintained their ethnic identity in Chinese communities and "Chinatowns" everywhere.

Over centuries, each of the different ethnic regions physically and philosophically encountered the medicine of China, introduced by Chinese traders and military expeditions, as well as these millions of "overseas Chinese" settlers. Each ethnic group made its own contribution to the knowledge and practices introduced from Chinese medicine, based upon its own unique herbal and plant resources, as well as traditional healers.

Two of the Chinese medical concepts common throughout the region are (1) the *celestial origins* of medical knowledge and healing practices, and (2) the key to all life, health, and healing is *vital energy* that influences all aspects of medical practice. Combining these concepts of celestial origins and vital energy, we may identify this synergy as the spiritual component to the "mind–body connection" commonly identified in Asian medical systems (see Micozzi 2011). In Chinese medicine, *qi* has a meaning, not as a static form that stands alone, but as an entity that *flows, in relation to other elements of the cosmos*. This property may be likened to the waterways of ancient Chinese civilization, a key feature of irrigation agriculture, the construction and maintenance of which was critical to the development of Chinese civilization, culture, and character. Like water, it is flow that brings *vital energy* to the organs and channels (meridians) it traverses or inhabits. The flow and cultivation of *qi*, like the flow of water for cultivation of the land, is critical to wellbeing. Q*i* is commonly encountered in Chinese, reflecting its broad application in everyday usage in words that describe atmosphere, emotion, environment, feeling, and flavor (for example the word *ki* is used in Japan; see Chapter 8).

In the West *qi* has been translated to refer to the flow of energy, spirit, or breath that animates living entities. Ancient Chinese ideograms depicted the term with three strokes to symbolize cloudlike vapor, as when the breath is vaporized and crystallized, as can be seen on a cold day. During the Northern Song Dynasty (960–1127 CE) the character for *qi* was elaborated to include four strokes (气), above the character for rice (米), and this form (氣) continues to be used in classical Chinese. This representation denotes a metabolic quality of steam/vapor rising over rice/food.

This character for rice (*fan*) means the specific grain, rice, but also has a more generic meaning of food or foodstuff, as in its use in *fan djian*, literally "rice hall," for restaurant or eating place. This meaning implies the broader metabolic context of this concept of vital energy. Contemporary Chinese *pinyin* has simplified the term to the top four strokes (气), but without including the character beneath for rice.

Daoist texts, as early as 300 BCE, with later recordings on bamboo and silk documents, describe *qi* as an elemental force shaping the *cosmos*, as well as the individual human body and personality. Q*i* may manifest itself in many forms on a spectrum from refined and immaterial, to condensed and heavy. It can be cultivated by the individual through breathing and physical movements (*qi gong*), and can be influenced and manipulated by Chinese medical practices such as acupuncture. In Daoism, "Breathing for life" is a practice for accessing *qi* as an energetic force. Encounters with *qi* can be quite subjective, but the overall experience of *qi* as energy and generative force shows it as essential to life itself.

Qi became essential for understanding the body and for medical practice in *East Asia*, beginning with Chinese medicine and its subsequent translation into *Korean* and *Japanese* forms of medicine. These three medical systems explicitly refer to *qi* (*gi* or *ki*) as a form of energy that shapes all entities in the cosmos. Consideration of ideas of vital healing in *Ayurveda*, *Unani* (Greco-Islamic), and *Tibetan* medicines bear resemblance to *qi* energy healing (see Micozzi 2011).

The Spiritual Pivot

Early references to *qi* in ancient Chinese medical texts are expressed in terms of vapor. Study of these medical texts has been interpreted to show that the concepts of "life nurturance" and "transformative practices" were integrated with earlier ideas of *yangsheng* ("nurturing generation") through *breath cultivation* and *meditation*. These practices are also common to many Asian traditions and seen as integral to one another.

These early concepts of *qi* were in use prior to the more formal definitions of *qi* expressed in later classic Chinese medical texts, such as the *Huangdi Neijing*, which consists of two classic texts (the *Suwen*, 素問, or *Basic Questions*, and *Lingshu*, 靈樞, *Spiritual Pivot*). These chapters consist of a dialogue or series of questions between the Yellow Emperor, *Huangdi*, and his ministers, including *Qi Bo*. The *Suwen* in translation identifies *qi* as essential to the human body. It is frequently used together with the term for blood (*xue*, 血), and a systematic hierarchy among bodily substances shows that wherever *qi* flows, so does blood.

The *Suwen* also discusses the systematic, hierarchical relations of the Five Organs (*zang*, 臟)—the heart (*xin*, 心), spleen (*pi*, 脾), lung (*Fei*, 肺), kidney (*shen*, 腎), and liver (*gan*, 肝)—and how each of these entities houses different forms of *qi*. These systemic, systematic relations are also known as the *Five Phases* (*wu xing*, 五行) and *Six Qi* (*liu qi*, 六氣). The Five Organs also facilitate close functional relations among *qi* and emotional states which may be likened to the four humors of medieval Europe:

1. With anger (choleric, or yellow bile), *qi* rises.

2. With happiness (phlegmatic, or phlegm), *qi* is relaxed.

3. With sadness (melancholic, or black bile), *qi* dissipates.

4. With fear (sanguine, or blood), *qi* moves down.

In the *Suwen*, *qi* refers to a range of emotional and mind–body states as well as pathological conditions due to disease. In other parts of the *Suwen*, essential (*ying*, 營) *qi* and defensive (*wei*, 衛) *qi* are paired opposites. These forms reflect the *qi* obtained from food and water that can either move within a vessel (*ying qi*) or within the skin (*wei qi*). Movements of *qi* are determinants of health, while the cessation of movement means disease or death. Thus, movement or circulation is central to the concept of *qi* in health and illness. The original text of the *Lingshu*, the second part of the *Huangdi Neijing*, no longer exists, and available translations are from later compilations completed in the twelfth century. The *Lingshu* (*Spiritual Pivot*), also called the *Canon of Acupuncture*, addresses the meridians (*jingluo*, 經絡) or channels for the flow and circulation of *qi*, and the acupuncture points (*zhenxue*, 針穴), through which *qi* enters and leaves the body. The flow or movement of *qi* within the body can be influenced by acupuncture techniques.

Beyond the analogies of the flow of *qi* for cultivation of a healthy body with the flow of water for cultivation of the land through irrigation agriculture, there is further correlation of bodily channels and organs to ministerial positions, functions and government organizations that indicate the close correspondences among the human body and the collective state in Chinese cosmology. The flow of *qi* in the universe and within the human mind–body influences both political structure and divine, rightful rule, so that the greater cosmological order reflected ancient Chinese bureaucracy and monarchy. The notion that knowledge about the technologies of civilization, such as agriculture, irrigation, and medicine, flowed to humans from celestial heavenly sources further enforced the idea of divine, rightful rule.

Today, one hundred years after the "Last Emperor" as the son of heaven, the health of Chinese society with extended family and other social kinship networks, is still seen in terms of the circulation and movement of vital *qi*. However, the impact of the largest social experiment in human history—that is, limiting the modern Chinese family to one child, and eliminating the kinship network of brothers/sisters, aunts/uncles, nieces/nephews—has yet to be reckoned with in relation to this fundamental social organization.

Transmission of energy

Through these classical texts, fundamental concepts about the cosmos, emanating from celestial revelations, became integral to medical theories about the body and appropriate treatment. These concepts *traveled widely* as the introduction of Chinese medicine took place wherever exchange occurred throughout Greater China and beyond. As traders, nomads, and emissaries traversed the Silk Routes, Chinese medical texts and medicinal herbs provided tangible products for these circuits and exchanges of trade. Today China's traditional medicine is practiced, in various forms, all over the world (see Part IV). In some places its practice follows the contemporary conventional formulation of traditional Chinese medicine (TCM, or *zhong yi*—see 'Note to the reader' below). Elsewhere it is fundamentally influenced by local custom, preference, or traditional interpretations. The spread of Chinese medicine to other regions in Asia traveled by multiple paths through official delegations, medicinal herb traders, spiritual pilgrims, and itinerant healers—as well as permanent migrations of "overseas Chinese." The presence of Chinese medical theory and practice within healing traditions can be seen across present-day *East* and *Southeast Asia*, *Central Asia*, and *South Asia*. While diverse, *qi* in its multiple forms can be seen to inform these different manifestations of medical practice.

Chinese medicine and the concept of *qi* had reached the Southern and Central Asian regions where other ancient systems of medicine (*Ayurveda, Sufism, Unani*) were already being practiced. Energetic healing is central to these traditional systems of healing as well. The concept of the flow of energy within a body as a source of vitality is shared by Asian medical systems. Regional and local ethnomedical *knowledge of medicinal plants and herbs* was also fundamental to developing diverse, effective traditions of medical practice throughout South, East, and Southeast Asia.

This book presents the two core ideas of *celestial origins* and *vital healing* in the traditional medicine of China in Part I. Part II describes the traditional medicines of East Asia, and Part III, Southeast Asia, and the influences that can be seen as part of Greater China. Part IV considers (1) the global influence and practice of Chinese medicine, as one of only two truly worldwide systems of medicine today—the other being our own widely traveled modern western biomedicine, (2) its influences in the West, and (3) its role as one of the leaders of the global integration of traditional medical practices and resources into the modern world of global healthcare. Finally, in the Appendices, we give you the reader some simple guidelines on using the time-tested, readily-available, and easy-to-use remedies from China and Southeast Asia that are effective for a wide range of modern ailments as a benefit for your own health. Consistent with the tenets of Chinese medicine and nutrition, here is food (and medicine) for the body and mind.

Note to the reader

Chinese medicine is often referred to as traditional Chinese medicine (TCM) in Western societies, while in Chinese it is simply called *zhong yi* (Chinese medicine). The term TCM suggests a long history over five thousand years where theories and practices descended from a clear lineage of knowledge. However, this view is far from the truth, as TCM is specifically a formulation of post-1947 Communist China wherein Chairman Mao Tse Tung (Zedong) attempted to recover knowledge, and provide medical care, from the "great treasure house" of Chinese medicine, in the absence of modern westernized medicine. This book identifies the earlier medical theories as ancient, "classic," or "pre-modern" Chinese medicine, and the contemporary forms since 1950 as "TCM." The ancient form is characterized by a diversity that encompasses every aspect of organization and practice, from theory and diagnosis to prognosis, therapeutics, and the social organization of health care. By contrast, TCM became systematized during the 1950s in mainland China with TCM colleges, publications and medical texts, clinical and laboratory research, licensing practices, and standardization of knowledge. The institutional formulation of TCM as a state system of healthcare attempted to transform Chinese medicine in China from multiple schools of thought and practice to a streamlined body of knowledge transmitted through state-published medical texts rather than through generations of individual practitioners. Worldwide, and back in China itself, multiple schools of practice persist, with growing numbers of individual practitioners from Chinatowns to University Medical Centers.

PART I

❧

China

Chapter 1

The World of
Chinese Medicine

Over 5000 years ago the people of the Yellow River Valley in
what is now China became organized as a cohesive society that
would come to permanently dominate the southeast quadrant
of the Asian continent and eventually extend its influence
thousands of miles to the east and to the south over successive
centuries.

Greater China

In the cultural history of East and Southeast Asia it is useful
to consider the concept of "Greater China," radiating outward
from the Yellow River Valley and encompassing the contiguous
areas of Manchuria, Korea, Japan, Indochina, the Malaysian
Peninsula, and the Indonesian Archipelago. This vast area
came under Chinese influence through mercantile and military
expansion in the long period between the earlier phase of
"Further India" and the later waves of Islamic influence in
much of this part of the globe.

The peoples of this Chinese civilization also would
eventually travel to every corner of the earth, taking their
traditional culture, including traditional medicine, and

spreading it around the globe. Today, together with modern Western biomedicine, it is one of only two forms of medicine that can be said to be available in virtually every urban setting in the world.

Conversely, when foreign cultures encountered the dominant Chinese civilization, they would usually be brought into the fold. A famous example is when the Mongol invader from the West, Genghis Khan, conquered China. Within two generations, his grandson Kublai Khan had become thoroughly "sinified"—that is, he proverbially became *more Chinese than the Chinese*. He even came to symbolize the prototypical Chinese Emperor in the eyes of eighteenth- and nineteenth-century Western literary figures such as Samuel Taylor Coleridge, who used Kublai Khan in his poem of the same name, as the symbol of oriental despotism, eroticism, exoticism and splendor, all at once. This type of depiction of China came to be understood as actually a Western image of China and the East, labeled *Orientalism* by Edward Said (1978, in his book of the same name) in the twentieth century.

Consistency in diversity

The ability of the Chinese to incorporate valuable new discoveries and ideas was at the same time central to maintaining the core of their culture and cosmology.

An important example of China encountering and incorporating new ideas was the influence of Gautama the Buddha from India, who traveled into China and profoundly influenced its cosmology and culture. The spiritual tradition of Buddhism came to exist side by side with Confucianism and Daoism, again illustrating the ability of Chinese civilization to accommodate and incorporate *diverse* traditions. An Emperor of the Ming Dynasty (1368–1644) wrote these lines:

> In my garden
> Side by side
> Native plants
> Foreign plants.

Beyond the boundaries of accommodation and assimilation, the Chinese made efforts to protect the purity of their culture and civilization and to keep out foreign "barbarians." Such efforts are dramatically illustrated by the huge project for the construction of the Great Wall (the only manmade artifact that can be seen from outer space). At places it is only 50 miles from Beijing (*Bei* northern, *jing* capital)—at *Ba Da Ling*, for example. While keeping out the Islamic influence of the Middle Asian Muslim hordes during the Middle Ages, the Chinese nonetheless picked up a few new ideas from the animal kingdom just beyond the Great Wall for the menu of classic Northern Chinese cuisine (such as duck and lamb), as well as for transportation (such as the camel), for the important trade route, "the Silk Road."

Later, when nineteenth-century Europeans were the potential colonizers, the Chinese created "cantonments" for each of the European powers, to keep them isolated and obstruct the flow of European "contagion" into the culture, in places such as Port Arthur, Hong Kong, and Macao. Finally, the descent of the Red Curtain after the 1947 Communist take-over was designed to keep foreign influence out, and perhaps just as much to keep Chinese in.

Accommodating and incorporating *diversity*, while maintaining a *consistent cosmology*, is also an important characteristic of Chinese medicine, and so new discoveries and ideas about medicine did not supplant the old ones—they were just accommodated alongside. As we will read in Chapter 5, for example, the ancient practice of Chinese herbal medicine was not supplanted by the later discovery of acupuncture; instead, the two co-exist in a common Chinese cosmology of medicine.

Celestial origins, legendary rulers

The ancient mythology of Chinese medicine attributes the birth of medicine to three legendary and semi-mythical emperors who might be called the "celestial trinity." The semi-mythical origins of these three kings are said to extend back in time nearly 5000 years. However, please keep in mind that, as we shall see, the written records only pick up the story much later. The first references to medical practices that begin to resemble Chinese medicine as we know it today, do not occur until the end of the third century BCE. Acupuncture first surfaces as a therapeutic method in the first century BCE. Some interpretations of the ancient archaeological evidence and texts seek to establish a greater antiquity for acupuncture by drawing inferences between ancient stone artifacts and modern acupuncture needles. In considering the manner in which Chinese medicine is constructed, none of these theories can be discarded.

In addition to their medical revelations, each of the celestial trinity is also credited with introducing many other useful practices into the world, placing medicine into a truly holistic context with the development of other critical aspects of Chinese civilization.

Fu Xi, the Ox Tamer (伏羲, circa 3000 BCE), celestial origins of medicine

Fu Xi, or the *Ox Tamer*, taught people how to *domesticate animals*. He also divined the *Ba Gua*, eight symbols that became the basis for the *I Ching*, or *Book of Changes*. When Fu Xi reveals celestial knowledge of domestication of the main Chinese beast of burden and engine for physical labor (the original and all-time "Year of the Ox"), he illustrates medicine as an intrinsic part of human society as well as part of the natural order.

Shen Nong, the Divine Husbandman (神農, circa 2750 BCE), origins of Chinese herbal medicine

Shen Nong, or the *Divine Husbandman*, also known as the *Fire Emperor*, is said to have lived from 2737 to 2697 BCE. He introduced *agriculture* to the world when he taught the Chinese people how to cultivate plants and raise livestock. Shen Nong, the channel for celestial knowledge on agronomy and agriculture, demonstrates that the breeding of animals and plants includes cultivation of plants for medicines as well as food.

This semi-mythical sequence of animal domestication ("ox taming"), followed by agriculture and raising livestock ("divine husbandry"), maps to modern archaeological interpretations of the development of complex civilizations in areas such as the Yellow River Valley, where peoples first kept nomadic herds of semi-domesticated animals on the move, then eventually settled down in fertile areas to raise animals and grow crops in one place.

As the originator of Chinese herbal medicine, Shen Nong learned the therapeutic properties of herbs and other substances by tasting them. Later authors would attribute their own works to Shen Nong to indicate the antiquity and importance of their texts. A good example of this tradition is *The Divine Husbandman's Classic of the Materia Medica* (*Shen Nong Ben Cao Jing*), which was probably written in 220 CE and reconstructed in 500 CE by Tao Hong Jing. When it comes to Chinese antiquity, it is never easy to separate legend from fact, but all historical evidence points to the truly ancient character of herbal medicine in China, so it is appropriate that Shen Nong is considered its originator. This "Classic of Shen Nong" is not a treatise on ancient medical theory but a simple compilation of plant and other material substances and their influences on the body.

Huang Di, the Yellow Emperor (黃帝, circa 2650 BCE), origins of acupuncture and qi manipulation

Huang Di introduced a more spiritual, "heavenly," and less "earthy" (literally, likened to the roots and parts of medicinal plants) approach to balancing vitality, or *qi*, through application of acupuncture. This new method does not use material sources and substances, such as medicinal plants, and is literally "immaterial," allowing more direct access to the spiritual, celestial, aspects of healing—thus gaining the attribution, the "Spiritual Pivot." Today Huang Di is perhaps the most generally known of the three legendary emperors. Bringing his people wisdom gained from *visiting in the celestial realm of the immortals*, this "Father of the Chinese Nation" is credited with introducing the art of writing, the techniques for making wooden houses, boats, carts, bows and arrows, silk, and ceramics, as well as the practice of traditional Chinese medicine. In our archaeological sequence, this stage represents the later development of complex civilization, where further social organization was required—for example, for irrigation and controlling floods, among peoples who had settled down to raise crops and livestock.

The Yellow Emperor's Inner Classic (*Huangdi Neijing*) is the first document in which traditional Chinese medicine was described in a form familiar today. The text is divided into two books: *Simple Questions* (*Suwen*) is concerned with medical theory, such as the principles of *yin and yang* (paired opposites in dynamic equilibrium, which help define the nature of life), *the Five Phases* (which relate to dynamic processes in the body), and the effects of the seasons; *The Spiritual Axis* or *Spiritual Pivot* (*Ling Shu*) deals predominantly with acupuncture and moxibustion.

Like *The Divine Husbandman's Classic of the Materia Medica*, *The Yellow Emperor's Inner Classic* was not written by the emperor himself but was compiled long after his death, probably around 100 BCE. *The Yellow Emperor's Inner Classic* is still revered in modern times, both for its legendary context and for its medical contributions to Chinese culture. The text is written as a series of dialogues between the Emperor and his ministers, including the famous Qi Bo, whose excitement about the "new" treatment of acupuncture resonates down through the centuries until today. He describes to the Emperor that acupuncture represents a more "heavenly," or celestial, spiritual approach to healing that does not require the use of the older, dirty, smelly and often bad-tasting formulations of roots, barks and leaves of medicinal plants. Debates over the effectiveness and appropriateness of acupuncture in comparison with herbal remedies continue among Chinese practitioners to this day.

The celestial knowledge revealed to these three emperors, as recorded today, was recovered on materials ranging from silk documents excavated from the *Ma Wang Dui* Han tombs (168 BCE or earlier) to widely translated works such as the *Shen Nong Bencaojing* (神農本草經, *Divine Farmer's Materia Medica*) and the *Huangdi Neijing* (黃帝內經, *Yellow Emperor's Classic of Internal Medicine*, or *The Yellow Emperor's Inner Classic*).

Diversity, diffusion, and dissemination

While these legendary celestial origins remain diverse, with iconic texts, notable practitioners, and concepts that date back millennia, these medical systems are at the same time characterized as traditional or unchanging, consistent with Chinese cosmology. Each system of knowledge has significantly evolved often with the intervention of state institutions, originating in the pronouncements of these semi-mythical, demigod rulers of China as embodiments of the state (see the section on the Middle Kingdom on the following page). Furthermore, (1) travel of practitioners, (2) dissemination of classic textual translations, and (3) exchange and trade of the *materia medica* and pharmacopeia of Chinese remedies, across the whole of Asia, contributed to many manifestations of classic forms of medical knowledge.

The transmission of textual sources via translators depended in part on regional proximity, and on sharing the same written language, as was the case for ancient China, Japan, and Korea (where classical Chinese characters were in use until the fifteenth century CE). Another important factor in considering the spread of Chinese medicine is regional ethnomedical practices based on the use of *materia medica*, or effective herbal remedies common to geographical distributions where they grow. A common property embedded in all medical practices and materials is the role of *qi* or vital energy.

Celestial origins of vital energy

The two important aspects of Chinese medical cosmology that we address here are *vital energy* or *qi*, and the *celestial origins* of medical knowledge and practice.

First, *health* is a result of the proper *balance (yin/yang) of vital energy (qi)* in the body, and disease is a result of imbalance. The intervention of a Chinese medical practitioner helps to maintain or restore this balance of vital energy, thus maintaining or restoring health. Medicinal herbs, acupuncture, and physical manipulations (*tui na*) and exercises (*qi gong*) are different medical modalities for maintaining or restoring health through the balancing of vital energy. This balance of vital energy is the goal of all these modalities as different paths to the same end, metaphysically working in the same way.

As we have seen, another important aspect of Chinese medical cosmology is that the knowledge of these medical modalities is divinely revealed to humans from *celestial* sources. Since, as detailed above, every major aspect of Chinese medicine had its origin attributed to the writings and teachings of semi-mythical divine rulers in the line of Chinese Emperors, attribution to the heavens as the source of all human knowledge, which is channeled through demigod rulers, to mortal humans, forms the basis for Chinese civilization in general, as well as for health and healing. This is the source of the iconic Chinese characterization of its own civilization as representing the "Middle Kingdom," half way between heaven and earth. This concept is directly revealed in China's name for itself, *Zhong Guo*, literally "the land at the middle." The medicine of China is the medicine of this Middle Kingdom.

The Middle Kingdom

The metaphors of Chinese medicine provide a useful way of representing human functional anatomy and physiology. As an empirical system, Chinese medicine is tremendously sophisticated and nuanced in terms of devising treatments tailored to each individual and to his or her specific conditions.

While the heavens are the source of Chinese civilization, including medical knowledge, the political organization of China provides models for how the body functions. It is striking how, throughout all of Chinese medicine, anatomy, and pathology (see Chapter 4), terms relating to the political governance of society are used as metaphors for how the human body is regulated—that is, essentially as an analogy of human physiology.

This view is striking to the Western reader, since Western biomedicine uses the metaphor of a machine to describe functions of the human body: the mechanical model. While the human body has been used as a metaphor for the political governance of a human society—for example, by Thomas Hobbes in his famous treatise, *Leviathan* (1651)—we do not apply the reverse concept in Western medicine. *Leviathan* was in fact the body politic made manifest—a social body composed of cells of individual men, just as the human body is composed of individual cells.

Modern medicine is largely based on the premise that the body is essentially made up of populations of cells comprising tissues and organs which work together as regulated by physiology, just as populations of individuals make up societies and work together under political governance.

The Chinese use medical metaphors that describe human physiology in terms analogous with human socio-political organization. This utilization may relate to the preoccupation of Chinese civilization with the Emperor (as the *celestial* source of divine knowledge and wisdom), his mandarins at court, and the disseminated bureaucratic organization that provided the foundation for government administration of complex works, organizations and operations.

One of the great projects of the ancient Chinese civilization was the creation of canals or "waterways" for irrigation and for transportation. The requirements for organization of labor for such projects had a transactional relationship to the development of Chinese social organization and political control. These processes and relationships were described by Karl Wittfogel (1957) in the classic treatise *Oriental Despotism*. The inherent relations of the contours of Chinese society with (1) major public "infrastructure" projects, (2) the political organization of the Chinese government, and (3) the Chinese pictographic language needed and used for communications, result in a rich vocabulary of metaphors describing medical aspects of the human body as waterways, channels, etc., in the original Chinese language.

In most Western translations words like "meridians" for the acupuncture energy channels do not fully correspond to these more "fluid" Chinese metaphorical concepts.

A flood of knowledge

The *celestial origins* of knowledge, the concept of *vital energy*, and its character represented as *flow*, like water, are all illustrated in the following legend. The demigod Gun (鯀), grandson of Huang Di, the Yellow Emperor, failed to build dams to restrain the great floods that threatened China. In contrast, his son Da Yu (大禹), one of the forefathers of Daoism, managed to control the floods by opening natural pathways along geographical "lines of force" to drain the accumulated waters.

Controlling and directing the flow of water was seen as one of the first steps to a civilized world. In the *Lingshu*, the rivers and streams of *qi* within the body were originally compared to the natural waterways of China (compare the *nadi* of yoga and the sacred rivers of India). Once the analogy between *qi* channels and watercourses had been made, channeling of *qi* into routes around the body presented a significant way of bringing the body, like the waterways, under control. A similar process may have occurred with *qi gong*, whose traditional postures were probably developed from more spontaneous movements and breathing behavior.

The development and application of these ideas about the nature of health and healing are illustrated in the following two chapters, "The Dynasties of Chinese Medicine" and "The Concepts of Chinese Medicine."

Chapter 2

The Dynasties of Chinese Medicine

Little is actually known about the practice of medicine in China before 200 BCE. Ancient Chinese civilization started with nomadic tribes; originally scattered across Northern China, they eventually established permanent settlements and developed a social and political structure that became the Shang Dynasty (1766–1121 BCE). Ancestors were venerated and consulted on a variety of issues, including the cause of illness, through the use of oracle bones. The scapulae and other flat bones of early domesticated animals were boiled in large bronze pots (an achievement of early Chinese metallurgy that predated the more sophisticated technology that later allowed the manufacture of acupuncture needles). (See also Chapter 11.)

The Zhou overthrew the Shang and established one of China's longest-lasting dynasties (1122–221 BCE). The Zhou Dynasty continued many of the Shang practices, including consulting tortoiseshell oracles with the aid of *wu* (healer/priests). The *wu* acted as *celestial* intermediaries between the living and the dead, played important ritual roles in court activities and in divining the weather, and were called upon to combat demons that caused illness. One of the *wu*'s activities— chasing evil spirits away from towns and homes with spears—

may have become transferred to the human body itself, leading to the practice of acupuncture.

Toward the close of the Zhou Dynasty came a time of violent political strife and social upheaval known as the Warring States period. This era saw the emergence of two philosophers, Kong Fu Zi (*Confucianism*) and Lao Zi (*Daoism*), whose ideas about social and natural order were to have a lasting impact on Chinese culture, together with the influences of Prince Gautama the Buddha (*Buddhism*) from India. In medicine also a sense of natural order was emerging, and the human body was no longer seen as subject to the whims of spirits and demons, but rather as part of a coherent natural environment. Those ideas, rooted in the Zhou period, would blossom during the Han Dynasty.

The development of Chinese medical theory and practice

The Zhou Dynasty ended in 211 BCE after a period of confusion and political instability. The short-lived Qin Dynasty completed the first version of the Great Wall of China but disappeared soon afterwards. The Han Dynasty (206 BCE–219 CE) reunited the empire, created a stable aristocratic social order, expanded geographically and economically, and spread Chinese political influence throughout the adjacent peninsulas of *Korea* and *Vietnam* (*Indochina*). This dynasty was such a powerful force that today the Chinese people refer to themselves as "the Han." Great cultural developments took place during the Han, including integration of the Confucian doctrine, elements of yin–yang, and the *Five Phase Theory* (see Chapter 3). Written evidence first reveals the emergence of a medicine similar to the traditional Chinese medicine known in modern times.

The earliest medical literature that survives from that era consists of three texts discovered in tombs dating to 168 BCE, excavated at Ma Wang Dui in Hunan province. These texts discuss demons, magic, and the relation of yin and yang to the body. The writings present an early concept of energy channels in the body, but less developed than in later descriptions in *The Yellow Emperor's Inner Classic*. The Ma Wang Dui texts mention moxibustion and the use of heated stones, but they do not speak about acupuncture or specific points on the body, suggesting that the idea of acupuncture had not yet emerged at this time.

The Divine Husbandman's Classic of the Materia Medica (*Shen Nong Ben Cao*) appears during this era, presenting the first known example of what has become a very long line of formal descriptions of individual medicinal substances. This period also saw the publication of *The Yellow Emperor's Inner Classic*, with its detailed descriptions of medical theory and the use of acupuncture and moxibustion; its wisdom still guides the practice of traditional Chinese medicine today, and it is often quoted in contemporary medical texts. The *Classic of Difficult Issues* (*Nan Jing*) was compiled sometime during the first or second century CE, although its authorship is attributed to the legendary physician Bian Qu, who lived in the fifth century BCE. It marks a drastic shift in medical thinking away from magic elements and toward systematic organization of acupuncture theory and practice.

Such learned texts reflected the health care available to the elite, rather than the medical traditions of the general population. At that time, about 80 percent of Chinese people were illiterate farmers or peasants scratching out a bare subsistence and still using Stone Age technology. Their *ethnomedical* traditions were oral, locally oriented, and full of folk superstition, historical legend, and aspirations dominated by the hope of survival, carrying some of the ideas about ancestors and demons from the Shang and Zhou dynastic eras.

In 220 CE, after 30 years of strife and religious rebellion by Daoist sects, the Han Dynasty fell. After the Han there was another long period of division in China, although not as violent as the Warring States period at the end of the Zhou Dynasty. In 589 CE the Sui Dynasty reunified China, but it was soon succeeded by the Tang Dynasty (618–907 CE), considered by many to be the height of China's cultural development. The Tang Dynasty spread Greater China's influence as far as Korea, Japan, Mongolia, Central Asia, and Indochina (Vietnam). During this period, both Buddhism and Daoism strongly influenced medical thought.

Systematic Chinese medicine

By the time of the Sung Dynasty (960–1280 CE), the practice of medicine had become more specialized, and efforts were made to integrate past insights systematically. In 1027 CE, Wang Wei Yi designed and oversaw the casting of two bronze figures designed to illustrate the location of acupuncture points. The bronzes were pierced at the acupuncture points, covered with wax, and filled with water. When a medical student inserted a needle in the correct place, he pierced the wax over the hole and water dripped out, confirming that the needle had been correctly placed.

During the Sung Dynasty there was a huge advance in herbal therapeutics and the publication, under imperial decree, of several complete, illustrated herbalist texts. It was during this time that tastes and properties were assigned to herbs according to their yin or yang nature, and functions were assigned that were a result of the herb's nature and its ability to treat specific symptoms.

During the Sung, Jin, and Yuan dynasties (960–1368 CE) medical education became more formal, the Imperial College of Physicians was founded, and specialized medical thought and independent inquiry continued to develop. Much of what we recognize as Chinese medicine today stems from these three dynasties. Physicians of this period revisited some early theories and used them to develop new therapeutic approaches. They espoused the application of *Five Phase Theory* (*wu xing*), in which dynamic processes in the body are defined in terms of the *Five Phases*: *Earth, Metal, Water, Wood,* and *Fire.* Each of these phases is related to various organs of the body, the seasons, times of day, tastes, colors, vocalizations, and other factors (see Chapter 3). During these three dynasties, the Five Phases were studied most intensively in relation to seasonal influences and as a way of supplementing the body, purging it of evil influences, and enhancing yin.

Medicine in the Ming and Qing dynasties

From the fourteenth to the early twentieth century, Chinese physicians focused on lines of inquiry pursued in preceding dynasties. Some scholars consider the Ming Dynasty (1368–1644 CE) to be the peak of the cultural expression of *acupuncture and moxibustion* in China. In 1644 the Ming Dynasty fell to foreigners from *Manchuria* who founded the Qing Dynasty (1644–1911 CE). Folk herbal and medical traditions, as opposed to the ancient celestial wisdom of the three emperors, were collected, organized, and published for the first time in the Qing Dynasty. Political, economic, and social changes swept the land. The Chinese were forced to wear pigtails for the first time in their history, which the "Han" resented bitterly. New food crops, including maize (corn), sweet potatoes, peanuts, and potatoes, were imported from the Americas and Africa.

As cultural horizons broadened, the scope of medical inquiry expanded, shaking the classical underpinnings of Chinese medical thought. In 1822 acupuncture was formally eliminated from the Imperial Medical College. By the close of the Qing Dynasty in 1911, political and cultural institutions were in a state of decline. The scattered practitioners of traditional Chinese medicine found themselves increasingly under fire from the advocates of a new and modern China.

In contrast to the revealed wisdom of the three emperors, then in disrepute, folk remedies were finally extensively explored and recorded in the twentieth century under the guidance of the post-revolutionary government of China, resulting in such texts as *The Barefoot Doctor's Manual*.

Chapter 3

The Concepts of
Chinese Medicine

Down through the Dynasties of the last more than 2000 years, the philosophy of Chinese medicine springs from the concept of *yin and yang*. These two terms can be used to express the broadest philosophical concepts, as well as the most focused perceptions of the natural world. Yin and yang express the idea of opposing but complementary phenomena that exist in a state of dynamic equilibrium. The most ancient metaphor for this idea was the shady and sunny sides of a hill, the sunlit southern side representing yang, and the shaded northern side representing yin. They are part of one whole, but fundamentally different in character: on the bright, sunny, yang side, plants and animals are more prevalent, the air is drier, and the rocks are warm; on the dim, shaded, yin side, the air is moist and cool.

Yin and yang are always present simultaneously. As Lao Zi, the *Daoist* contemporary of Confucius, described, "The created universe carries the yin at its back and the yang in front." The paired opposites observed in the world give tangible expression to the otherwise incomprehensible Dao (the Way) of ancient Chinese thought. *The Book of Changes* (*I Ching*), which sought to explore the myriad manifestations of yin and yang, put it this way: "That which lets now the dark, now the light, appear is Dao."

Table 3.1 Yin and yang

Yang	Yin
Light	Dark
Heaven	Earth
Sun	Moon
Day	Night
Spring	Autumn
Summer	Winter
Hot	Cold
Male	Female
Fast	Slow
Up	Down
Outside	Inside
Fire	Water
Wood	Metal

The Yellow Emperor's Inner Classic was the first text to provide a comprehensive discussion of the medical application of yin and yang, and state that "yin and yang are the way of heaven and earth."

This text showed how yin and yang are used to correlate the body and other phenomena to the human experience of health and disease. It says, "As to the yin and yang of the human body, the outer part is yang and the inner part is yin. As to the trunk, the back is yang and the abdomen is yin. As to the organs, the bowels are yang, whereas the [other] viscera are yin. The liver, heart, spleen, lung, and kidney yin; the gallbladder, stomach, intestines, bladder, and triple burner [an organ known only in Asian medicine] are yang."

Yin and yang are used to express ideas not just about health and disease, but about the manner in which the entire *cosmos* is organized as well. These correspondences are similar to the classical and medieval European notions of the four humors. Summer is yang within yang; fall is yin within yang; the coldest, darkest, and most yin period, winter, is yin within yin; while spring, when the yang begins to emerge from the yin, is yang within yin. (See the following sections on the Five Phase correspondences.)

Yin and yang emphasize that reality is in a constant process of transformation and that all things are interconnected. A candle provides a useful analogy: if we consider the wax to be the yin aspect of the candle and the flame to be the yang, we can see how the yin nourishes and supports the yang, while the yang consumes the yin and, in doing so, burns brightly. When the wax is gone, so is the flame. Yin and yang exist interdependently.

The ancient Chinese understood human beings to have a nature and structure inseparable from yin and yang; and the same rules that guide the cosmos guide the human body. As in medieval and Renaissance Europe, the microcosm reflects the macrocosm (as illustrated in the works of Shakespeare, for example, and documented in E. M. W. Tillyard's classic twentieth-century study, *The Elizabethan World Picture*; see Tillyard 1959). It was said, "To follow [the laws of] yin and yang means life; to act contrary to [the laws of] yin and yang means death."

Within the traditional medical community of contemporary China, there is much debate over the actual nature of yin and yang. Some exponents of a more scientific, less traditional, perspective on Chinese medicine would like yin and yang to be used as concepts to organize phenomena. Others, who express a less modern perspective, emphatically state that yin and yang are actually tangible phenomena. While it is probably easiest for us to think about yin and yang as descriptive terms that help the Chinese physician to organize information, it should be remembered that in Chinese medicine, especially its medicinal substances, the yin and yang constituents of the body are considered material entities that can be reinforced by specific substances or actions.

The Five Phases: Earth, Metal, Water, Wood, and Fire

Another concept that has played a significant role in the development of Chinese medicine is that of the *Five Phases or processes (wu xing)*: *Earth, Metal, Water, Wood,* and *Fire*. In Chinese, *wu* means "five" and *xing* expresses the idea of movement, of going. For a period of time, the *wu xing* was translated as "the five elements." This translation conveys little of the dynamism of the Chinese concept, instead focusing on the apparent similarities between *wu xing* and the elements of medieval European alchemy. *Wu xing* may include the implication of material elements, but, in general, the term "Five Phases" better addresses the dynamic relations among phenomena that are organized in terms of these interconnected phases. This philosophy can cover almost every aspect of natural phenomena in the cosmos, from bodily organs to the weather.

The Five Phase Theory: constituents, organs, and powers

The human body is like an ecological system. As yin and yang divide the cosmos into two polar forces, five primordial powers differentiate all vital activity as progressing through Five Phases that correspond to the seasons in nature.

The body can be seen as a garden in this human landscape, encompassing the five primal forces in nature, which in turn correspond to the sequence of the seasons:

- Fire—yang—summer.
- Earth—yang and yin in balance—intervals between seasons.
- Metal—yin within yang—autumn.
- Water—yin—winter.
- Wood—yang within yin—spring.

The cycle of human life also corresponds to the seasons of nature:

- Water phase (yin)—gestation—*in utero.*
- Wood phase—birth—new life comes forth.
- Fire phase (yang)—maturation—adulthood.
- Metal phase—aging.
- Earth phase—interval between these stages.
- Water phase—again—death.

While the Five Phase elements correspond to the seasons in the environment (*macrocosm*), five functional systems, or organ networks, govern particular mental faculties, physiological activities, and tissues of the human body (*microcosm*):

- Water—Kidney.
- Fire—Heart.
- Wood—Liver.
- Metal—Lung.
- Earth—Spleen.

These organ networks generate and regulate the body's constituents:

- Blood—*nourishes*—gives solidity to the shape created by Qi; connective tissue.
- Essence—*provides foundation*—fundamental origin (ovum, sperm); genes, DNA.
- Moisture—*lubricates*—fluids: digestive, joints, eyes, cerebro-spinal fluid; buffers body.
- Qi—*moves*—vital force, flow, giving shape ("keeping it together"); adaptation.
- Shen—*embodies*—organizing force of the self, immaterial (yang); body–mind–spirit.

Blood, by itself, is inert, passive, thick, and, accordingly, has a tendency to stagnate, pool and congeal (clot). *Qi* is active and warms and moves the blood. *Qi* by itself has no material expression and no source for renewal. Providing the material basis, blood links *qi* with physical form. Blood is said to be the mother of *qi*, and where *qi* goes, blood flows.

Likewise, we can relate the body's ecology to that of nature and the cosmos:

- Shen—Heavens—integrative consciousness of body–mind–spirit, self-awareness.
- Qi—Air—animating force in all living processes, manifested as human activity.
- Moisture—Inner Sea—liquid medium that nurtures and lubricates interfaces.
- Blood—Soil—substances and structures of the body, repository of mental images.
- Essence—Earth/seeds—foundations and phenotypic expressions of basic identity.

Each organ network embodies a set of functions, psychological as well as physiological, corresponding to channels of influence, emotional states, sensory activity, as well as specific tissues. While they are assigned to a named anatomical structure, they are not fixed in location:

- Fire—Heart—envelops *Shen*, propels *Blood*, perception, and intuition.
- Metal—Lung—governs respiration, circulation of *Qi*, subconscious, defenses.
- Earth—Spleen—takes in nutrients, supplies *Moisture*, thought, and memory.
- Wood—Liver—governs *Blood*, circulating *Qi*, judgment, and temperament.
- Water—Kidney—stores *Essence*, instincts, impulses, will, and wisdom.

Physical processes are not limited to the body, and feelings and thoughts are not assigned to the brain. Each of five networks influences and regulates a set of both bodily and mental activities and processes.

As in the association with the seasons of nature, the Five Phases interact with each other according to countervailing sequences of generation and restraint, proliferation and limitation, through which balance is maintained. *Sheng* is the supporting sequence for generation and proliferation, and *Ke* is the restraining sequence for limitation. Each phase gives birth to the succeeding phase in the Sheng sequence, and each establishes limits on another in the Ke sequence, all in a cycle.

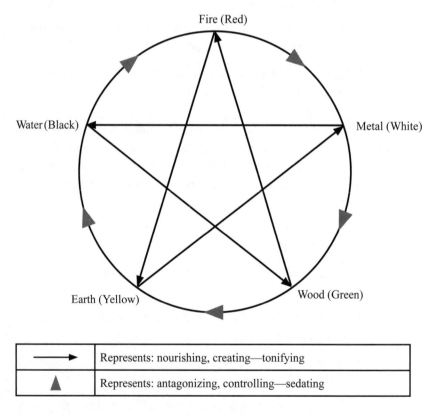

| → | Represents: nourishing, creating—tonifying |
| ▲ | Represents: antagonizing, controlling—sedating |

Figure 3.1 The five elements: nourishing and antagonizing relationships
Source: Repeti 2011

- *Sheng* supporting sequence:
  - ° Fire/Heart supports Earth/Spleen supports Metal/Lung supports Water/Kidney supports Wood/Liver supports Fire/Heart...and so the cycle continues.
  - ° Corresponding to the elements of nature, Water nourishes Wood, Wood feeds Fire, Fire generates Earth, Earth gives rise to Metal, Metal vitalizes Water.
- *Ke* restraining sequence:
  - ° Fire/Heart controls Metal/Lung controls Wood/Liver controls Earth/Spleen controls Water/Kidney controls Fire/Heart...and continue.
  - ° In nature, Water quenches Fire, Fire tempers Metal, Metal restrains Wood, Wood covers Earth, Earth dams Water.

Deficiency diseases usually develop along the Sheng sequence. Diseases of excess often advance from one organ network to another on the Ke sequence. The gravity of a disease is assessed by how far along each of the sequences it has progressed, and consequently, how many organ networks are effected.

Balancing vital energy

The crucial concept of *qi* or vital energy relates to the idea that the body is pervaded by subtle material and mobile influences that cause most physiological functions and maintain the health and vitality of the individual. This idea is not common to biomedical thinking about the body, and it is not easy for Westerners to grasp it. The common translation of *qi* as "energy" conceals its distinctly material attributes. While energy is defined as the capacity of a system to do work, the character of *qi* extends considerably further.

The Chinese character for *qi*, as we have seen, is traditionally composed of two radicals (word elements): the radical that symbolizes breath or rising vapor is placed above the radical for rice. *Qi* is linked with the concept of "vapors arising from food," and while the concept of *qi* broadened over time, it never lost its distinctly material aspect. To make the concept even more confusing, some phenomena labeled as *qi* do not fit conventional definitions of either substance or matter. The phrase "finest matter influences" or even just "influences" may offer a better translation. It is easy to see why many prefer to leave the term *qi* untranslated.

The idea of *qi* is extremely broad, encompassing almost every variety of natural phenomena. There are many different types of *qi* in the body, depending on its source, location, and function. There has been much ancient and modern debate, but in general, *qi* is seen as having the functions of activation, warming, defense, transformation, and containment.

The *qi* concept is important to many aspects of Chinese medicine. Organ and channel *qi* are influenced by *acupuncture*; in fact, one characteristic feature of acupuncture treatment is the sensation of "obtaining the qi." *Qi gong* is a general term for the many systems of meditation, exercise, and therapeutics anchored in the concept of mobilizing and regulating the movement of *qi* in the body. *Qi* is sometimes compared to wind captured in a sail; one cannot observe the wind directly, but can infer its presence as it fills the sail. In a similar fashion, movements of the body and the movement of substances within the body are all signs of the action of *qi*.

For instance, in accordance with the Five Phase system, *qi* conveys blood throughout the body; blood flows through the body with the *qi*. Blood is understood to have a slightly broader and less definite range of actions in Chinese medicine than it does in biomedicine. Generally, blood is seen as nourishing the body; it is produced by the construction *qi*, which in turn is derived from food and water. Within the body, *qi* and blood are said to be as closely linked as are a person and his or her own shadow. This relation is expressed by the Chinese saying, "*Qi* is the commander of blood, and blood is the mother of *qi*," using the social-political metaphors common to Chinese medicine.

Body fluids—thin and viscous substances that serve to moisten and lubricate the body—can be conceptually separated into humor and liquid. Humor is thick and related to the body's organs; among its functions is the lubrication of the joints. Liquid is thin and is responsible for moistening the surface areas of the body, including the skin, eyes, and mouth. In relation to *qi*, blood and fluids constitute the yin aspects of the body.

Qi, essence, and spirit

Qi, *essence*, and *spirit* are known in Chinese medicine as "the three treasures." Essence is the gift of one's parents (like genes), and spirit is the *celestial* gift of heaven.

Essence is the most fundamental source of human physiological processes, of the bodily reserves that support human life, and of the actual reproductive substances of the body. It must be replenished by food and rest.

Spirit is the alert and radiant aspect of human life. We see it in the luster of the eyes and face in a healthy person, as well as in that person's ability to think and respond appropriately to the world around us. The idea expressed by spirit, or *shen*, encompasses consciousness and healthy mental and physical function.

This connection reflects the concept that mind and body are not separated, but fully interactive in a complex and dynamic way. Mental and emotional experiences impact the body, and vice versa. Aspects of human experience that are understood as predominantly mental in a biomedical frame of reference are linked to specific organs in Chinese medicine—for example, anger is related to the liver, thought to the spleen, and joy to the heart. These correspondences guide the application of balancing methods used for treatment in acupuncture, *tui na*, reflexology, *qi gong*, and herbalism, as we shall see in the chapters that follow.

Choices in Chinese medical concepts

Since there are many choices in Chinese medical concepts and approaches to be used for both the Chinese and the Western patient, there are many pathways for a traditional Chinese practitioner to learn and practice from among these different concepts. The medicine that works best is often the modality that best meets our cultural expectations and "comfort zone." Understanding acupuncture and other traditional forms of healing begins with the unique cultural environment in which it has been developing for thousands of years.

Medicine is a human endeavor, and as such it is shaped by human concerns, including economics, politics, and culture. A medical scientist or a physician might perceive medicine as a steady march from ignorance to light, but these are typically revisionist histories. In the practice of medicine, ideology, belief, convenience, and even simple ignorance have probably had a greater influence than rationality.

Take, for instance, the choice of how to conduct a medical procedure. An example is the case of a Chinese patient who chose traditional herbal medicine to manage painful and debilitating kidney stones. Although the treatment ultimately took care of his problem, his choice was less medically based than career-driven. He knew that if he had undergone surgery, he would have been classified as an invalid on his work papers and therefore barred from advancement in his job. Institutions are as culturally biased as are individuals. (There remain hospitals which close their doors to the practice of acupuncture, despite the fact that acupuncturists are licensed medical practitioners and their services are routinely requested by hospital patients.) In each instance, health care choices primarily involved cultural considerations, not medical ones.

Our own definitions of medicine, even of the human body and how it works, are profoundly affected by culture; we carry with us firmly entrenched expectations about our own and other healing systems. For instance, we tend to envision Chinese herbal medicine as a gentle therapy using benign ingredients, overlooking the fact that it also incorporates highly toxic substances and drastic purgative therapies. We are selective in how we explore other medicines. Naturalistic and rational elements intrigue us, but unfamiliar elements tend to make us uncomfortable—such as the idea that medical knowledge is revealed from celestial sources to divine rulers—so we tend to ignore them.

When we encounter new ideas, we often like to think about them in familiar terms. This tendency can be seen in the use of the word "energy" to express the idea of *qi*, or the word "sedation" as a translation for the therapeutic method of draining "evil influences" from channels in the body. Neither energy nor sedation has much to do with the concepts that underlie *qi* and draining; however, these terms are more familiar to us and make Chinese medicine more accessible.

Unfortunately, these handy translations are inaccurate and can obscure the breadth and depth of meaning in these terms. We have a tendency to think of Chinese medicine as a monolithic structure that has remained essentially unchanged since its origins, which, if legend is to be believed, reach back 5000 years. Instead, as we have seen, Chinese medicine includes a tremendously diverse body of knowledge. It is extremely tempting for Westerners to expect medical systems to be possessed of an internal logic that reconciles all of their elements. Although many aspects of Chinese medicine fit together with complete consistency, others appear to be quite contradictory. This trait leads us to what has probably been the most important aspect in understanding Chinese medicine throughout its history: certain medical practices might have been relegated to the attic, but they remain available if needed.

A striking example is the work of Zhang Zhong Jing (142–220 CE), whose system of diagnosis and therapy did not attract much attention during his lifetime but became highly influential centuries after his death. Later Chinese medical practitioners believed his theory to be incomplete and broadened its perspective, but his theories, and the new theories that emerged in response to them, are still important to the contemporary Chinese clinician. In the West, an incomplete theory is rejected and then disappears. In the history of Chinese medicine, theories, practices, and concepts may fade away, but they do not entirely vanish. A new theory can exist beside the one that it sought to replace. The clinician can choose to apply the perspective that he or she feels is most appropriate. In this way, conflicting concepts, systems of diagnosis, and treatments have continued to exist side by side over many centuries.

The logic of inconsistency

> You say I am inconsistent. Then, I am
>   inconsistent.
> I am large. I contain multitudes.

> (Walt Whitman)

Where Western biomedicine believes all theories are proved either right or wrong, and should accordingly be retained or eliminated, Chinese medicine embraces multiple theories, like the yin yang character of all things, knowing that each may prove its utility when the right circumstances arise.

Even in modern China, where the sheer volume of information and the size of the population make it necessary to teach a standard curriculum to thousands of students each year, this tolerance for varying clinical perspectives continues. There are, for instance, herbal physicians known as "minor bupleurum decoction (*Xiao Chai Hu Tang*) doctors" because their prescriptions are organized around *one herbal medicinal* formula from the *Treatise on Cold Damage* (*Shang Han Lun*), an early text on diagnosis and herbal therapy written during the Han Dynasty (206 BCE–220 CE). There also are *herbal physicians* who reject traditional formulas entirely and use contemporary biomedical research on the Chinese pharmacopoeia to organize their prescriptions.

Within *acupuncture*, there are practitioners whose clinical focus might be dedicated almost entirely to only six acupuncture points and who now use CT scans to plan interventions. At the same time, two floors down in the same hospital, physicians may base their selection of acupuncture points on obscure and complex aspects of traditional calendars and systems such as the "Magic Turtle."

In China, while a practitioner might be limited to the use of only *six acupuncture points*, in the U.S., a licensed medical doctor can become an acupuncturist with only *six weeks of training*; and in Chinatowns around the world, practitioners must have *six generations* in their lineage in order to be trusted.

Any form or choice of health care modality works best when it meets the cultural expectations of the recipient (which is not to say that the powerful effects of the modalities are attributable merely to the "placebo effect"). Practitioners of Chinese medicine discovered aspects of human physiology that are not utilized in Western biomedicine. The fact that they are expressed in terms that are consistent with Chinese views of the cosmos and conceptualizations of how medical knowledge originates from celestial sources does not make them any less valid than Western "scientific" constructs in terms of the empirical evidence for their effectiveness.

Chapter 4

The Body of Chinese Medicine

Anatomy and physiology

The ancient Chinese did not focus on anatomical or pathological dissection as a primary way of understanding the body, and so their definitions of the organs were made according to function rather than physical structure. The physician of Chinese medicine encounters a body in which 12 organs function. These organs are divided into the viscera, which include six *Zang* or solid organs—heart, lungs, liver, spleen, kidneys, and pericardium (sac of membranes around the heart)—and the bowels, which include six *Fu* or hollow organs—the small intestine, large intestine, gallbladder, stomach, urinary bladder, and the "triple burner" (*san jiao*). Chinese and Western definitions of these organs and their functions match in many ways, but there are key differences as well. For instance, in the Chinese system, the liver is said to store blood and distribute it to the extremities as needed, and the spleen is understood as an organ of digestion.

The circulation and elimination of fluids was observed and attributed to an organ that is said to have a name, but no form; this is the "triple burner" mentioned above. It is considered to be either the combined expression of the activity of other organs in the body or a group of spaces in the body. The "triple burner" has always been surrounded by debate within Chinese medicine because it does not have a clear anatomical structure, only a physiological function.

The viscera and bowels are paired in what is known as the yin and yang, or interior/exterior relationship. The heart is linked with the small intestine, the spleen with the stomach, and so on. Each of the viscera—and each bowel—has an associated channel that runs through it, through the paired organ within the body, and across the body's surface, before connecting with the channel of the paired organ.

Historical evidence suggests that the idea of channels is more ancient than the idea of specific acupuncture points. Disagreements continue about the locations of specific points, and efforts have been made to systematize knowledge of them. Recent research in the People's Republic of China has led to the publication of a number of texts dedicated to reconciling historical perspectives, terminology, and anatomic questions about acupuncture points. At this time, there are understood to be 12 primary channels and eight extraordinary channels. *Qi* is understood to flow in these channels, making a rhythmic circuit.

Along the pathways of 14 of these channels (the 12 regular channels and two of the extraordinary channels) lie 361 specific points. In addition, a large number of "extra" points have been derived from clinical experience, but are not traditionally considered part of the major channel systems. Beyond this formulation, various individual acupuncture theories suggest still other points. There are also local microsystems of acupuncture points on the *ear* (*auricular acupuncture*—see Chapter 6), *scalp, hand, foot* (*corresponding to reflexology*—see Chapter 7), and other areas of the body.

Acupuncture points are most often located where a gentle and sensitive hand, with slight pressure on the skin surface, detects a small depression or downward slope. Points exist at the margins or bellies of muscles, in between bones, and over distinctive bony features that can be detected through the skin. Methods used to find acupuncture points vary. In general, points are located by seeking anatomic landmarks (considered the most reliable), by proportionally measuring the body, or by using finger measurements.

As with *qi*, the actual term and usage of the Chinese expression that we translate as "point" is important. The character *xue*, which has been translated as point, literally means "hole" in Chinese, which may more accurately reflect the clinician's subjective experience of the acupuncture site. *Xue* are holes where the *qi* of the channels can be influenced by inserting a needle, or by other means, such as moxibustion. If you imagine the channel system as a vast internal waterway, with caves and springs punctuating its course, you will have a concept of the *xue*, or hole, that is not far from the way the Chinese thought of them for many centuries.

Holes, or points along the channels, have been categorized and organized in many ways. One of the oldest and most well known is a system of categories based on the idea of *shu*, or transport points. This system of point categories applies exclusively to points on the forearm and lower leg, which embody the image of *qi* welling gently forth from a mountainous source at the tips of fingers and toes, and gradually gaining strength and depth as it reaches the seas located at the elbow and knee joints.

What causes disease?

Ultimately, all illness is a disturbance of *qi* within the body. Its expression as a particular disorder displaying specific symptoms depends on the location of the disturbance. Three categories of disease causation are recognized: external, internal, and causes that are neither external nor internal.

The three causes of disease (san yin)

- External causes, or the "six evils": wind, cold, fire, damp, summer heat, and dryness.

- Internal causes, or internal damage by the seven affects: joy, anger, anxiety, thought, sorrow, fear, and fright.

- Non-external, non-internal causes: dietary irregularities, excessive sexual activity, trauma, parasites, and taxation fatigue (too much or too little activity).

The first category includes six influences that are distinctly environmental: wind, cold, fire, dampness, summer heat, and dryness. When they cause disease, these six influences are known as "evils." If the defense *qi* is not robust, or the correct *qi* is not strong, or if the evil is powerful, then the evil may enter the surface of the body and, under certain conditions, penetrate to the interior.

The nature of the evil and its impact on the body are understood through the observation of nature and of the body in illness. In this sense, the biomedical distinction between cause and disease is somewhat blurred in Chinese medical theory. For example, the evils of wind and cold are frequently implicated in the sudden onset of symptoms that are associated with the common cold: headache, pronounced aversion to cold, aching muscles and bones, fever, and a scratchy throat. *Wind* is expressed in the suddenness of the symptoms' onset and in their manifestation in the upper part of the body; *cold* is displayed in the pronounced aversion to cold and in aching muscles and bones. Whether the person had a specific encounter with a cold wind shortly before the onset of the symptoms is not particularly relevant. Although it is not unusual for people to announce that they have been out on a chilly and windy day prior to the onset of a cold, such exposure could easily result in signs of wind heat as well—that is, a less marked aversion to cold, a distinctly sore throat, and a dry mouth. The six evils are not the agents of specific diseases, but rather the agents of specific symptoms. These ideas developed in a setting where there was no means of investigating a bacterial or viral cause. Instead, careful observation of the body's response to disease provided the information necessary for treatment.

Each of the evils affects the body in a fashion similar to its behavior in the environment. The human body stands between heaven and earth, and is subject to the influences of both. Although these six evils are identified as environmental influences that attack the body's surface, it also is clearly understood they may occur within the body, causing internal disruption.

Internal damage by the *seven affects* relates to the way in which mental states can influence body processes. However, this statement implies a separation of mind and body that does not exist in Chinese medicine. Each of the seven affects can disturb the body if it is strongly or frequently expressed or repressed. As was mentioned in Chapter 3, each of the mental states—joy, anger, anxiety, thought, sorrow, fear, or fright—is related to a specific organ.

Non-external, non-internal causes encompass the origins of disease that do not arise specifically as a result of environmental influences or mental states. These include dietary irregularities, excessive sexual activity, taxation fatigue caused by overwork or extreme inactivity, trauma, and parasites. The role that most of these have in producing disease is obvious to us, with the exceptions of excessive sexual activity and taxation fatigue. Excessive sexual activity suggests the possibility that too frequent emission of semen by the male can cause illness. This can occur because semen is directly related to the concept of essence, which is considered to be vital to the body's function and difficult to replace. This category also includes possible damage to the essence through excessive childbearing, or bearing a child at too young or too old an age.

Taxation fatigue is an intriguing category which concerns the dangers of engaging in a variety of activities for a prolonged period of time. It includes both the idea of overexertion and the idea of excessive inactivity as possible causes of disease. All of the concepts included within taxation fatigue reflect the essential thought of Chinese medicine that moderation is the key to health. Lying down for prolonged periods damages the *qi*, and prolonged standing damages the bones. From the moment when the Yellow Emperor asks Qi Bo, in the *Classic of Internal Medicine*, why people now die before their time, and receives the answer that *balance*, *harmony*, and *moderation* are key, these images have informed Chinese medicine.

Qi Bo explains the orderly life of times past

In *The Yellow Emperor's Inner Classic*, the first book, "Simple Questions" begins with the Yellow Emperor asking his minister, Qi Bo, why life-spans are now so short, when in the past people lived close to one hundred years. Qi Bo explains that in the past people maintained an orderly life. "In ancient times those people who understood Dao [the Way] patterned themselves upon the yin and the yang, and they lived in harmony with the arts of *divination*."

Each of the causes of disease—from prosaic ones, such as dietary irregularities, to somewhat exotic notions, such as wind evil—disrupts the *balance* (of yang and yin) within the body and disrupts the free movement of *qi*. Learning the precise pattern of imbalance is the beginning of the diagnostic process.

Diagnosis

There are four main methods of diagnosis in Chinese medicine: *inspection*, *listening and smelling*, *inquiry*, and *palpation*. The fundamental goal is to collect information that reflects the status of mind–body processes, and then to analyze this information to determine how each process has been affected by a disorder.

- *Inspection* (*wang*) refers to the visual assessment of the patient, particularly the spirit, form and bearing; the head and face; and the substances excreted by the body. The color, shape, markings, and coating of the tongue are carefully inspected. In the case of a person who had been attacked by wind and cold, for instance, we would expect to see a moist tongue with a thin white coating, signaling the presence of cold. If heat were present, we might expect a dry mouth and a red tongue. The observation of the spirit, which is considered very important, relies on assessing the overall appearance of the patient, especially the eyes, the complexion, and the quality of the voice. Good spirit—even in the presence of serious illness—is thought to bode well for the patient.

- *Listening and smelling* (*wen*) indicates listening to the quality of speech, breath, and other sounds, as well as to being aware of the odors of breath, body, and excreta. As is the case with each aspect of diagnosis, Five Phase Theory can be incorporated into the assessment of the person's condition. Each phase and each pair of viscera and bowel has a corresponding vocalization and smell.

- *Inquiry*, the third method of diagnosis (which, like listening and smelling, is also known as *wen*), involves taking a comprehensive medical history. This process has been presented in many ways, but perhaps best known is the system of ten questions described by Zhang Jie Bin in the Ming Dynasty. The questions were presented as an outline of diagnostic inquiry and included asking the patient about sensations of hot and cold, perspiration, head and body, excreta, diet, chest, hearing, thirst, previous illnesses, and previous medications and their effects. For example, an inquiry of the hypothetical patient suffering from wind and cold symptoms would be likely to reveal an aversion to any sort of exposure to cold, along with headache, body aches, and an absence of thirst. Inquiry is considered critical to a good diagnosis. Although pulse diagnosis is sometimes regarded as a central feature of Chinese medicine and is rightly regarded as an art, it should not form the sole basis of a diagnosis.

- *Palpation* (*qie*), the fourth diagnostic method, involves pulse examination, general palpation of the body, and palpation of the acupuncture points. Pulse diagnosis offers a range of approaches and can provide a remarkable amount of information about the person's condition. The process of pulse diagnosis is carried out with the person in a calm state, sitting or lying down. The physician's fingers are placed on the radial arteries of the left and right wrists, approximately where a pulse is normally taken in Western medicine. There are three pulse positions, known as the inch, the bar, and the cubit. The *inch* position, which is nearest the wrist, indicates the status of the body above the diaphragm; the *bar* indicates the status of the body between the diaphragm and the navel; and the *cubit* indicates the status of the area below the navel. Beyond this simple conceptual structure (and variations in technique), each pulse position can be interpreted to shed light on the status of the various organs and channels. The pulse allows the clinician to feel the quality of the *qi* and blood at different locations in the body. Pulse qualities are organized on the basis of size, rate, depth, force, and volume of the pulse. The practitioner will recognize such pulse qualities as rough, slippery, or bowstring. The clinician with many years of experience can find great meaning in overall quality of the pulse and the variations in quality at certain positions. For instance, the hypothetical patient afflicted with a wind-cold evil might display a pulse that was floating and tight, signaling the presence of a cold evil on the surface of the body.

Once the practitioner of Chinese medicine has carried out the diagnostic processes, he or she must construct an appropriate image of the disease's configuration so that it can be addressed by effective therapy. Central to this process is the notion of *pattern identification* (*bian zheng*), the process of gathering signs and symptoms through the diagnostic process and using traditional theory to understand how fundamental substances of the body, the organs, and the channels have been affected.

The first step of pattern identification is localization of the disorder and the assessment of its essential nature, using the *eight principles* that are an expansion of yin and yang correspondences: *yin, yang, cold, hot, interior, exterior, vacuity* (sometimes translated as *deficiency*), and *repletion* (sometimes translated as *excess*). The *Five Phases* may also be used, alone or in conjunction with the yin and yang correspondences.

Like many other aspects of contemporary Chinese medicine, the eight principles originated in the Sung Dynasty (960–1280 CE). Kou Zong Shi proposed a structure that organized disease into eight essentials: cold, hot, interior, exterior, vacuity, repletion, evil *qi*, and right *qi*. These were improved upon in 1732, in the text *Awakening the Mind in Medical Studies* (*Yi Xue Xin Wu*). The original source was written, in the spirit of the times, to create a formal diagnostic structure for herbs that could be conceptually integrated with the ideas already in use for acupuncture. Today this formal structure is applied to both acupuncture and herbal medicine.

Say the hypothetical wind-cold patient came to us with these symptoms: a marked aversion to exposure to cold, headache, body aches, an absence of thirst, a moist tongue with a thin white coating, and a floating and tight pulse. In terms of the eight principles, this would be an *exterior, cold, repletion* pattern. The principles of yin and yang would not directly apply.

What does this mean? The eight principles serve fundamentally to localize a condition. When a Chinese physician says that a condition is *external*, he or she means that it has not yet penetrated beyond the skin and channels to the deeper parts of the body. In this case a *cold* condition betrays itself through the body's expression of cold signs. To say a condition is *replete* is to say that the evil attacking the body is strong.

Typically, the eight principles are the first step in developing a clear pattern identification, especially if there is organ involvement. The eight principles are the application of a yin and yang-based theoretical structure.

Chinese diagnosis often cannot be related to single biomedical disease. For example, viral hepatitis is associated with at least six distinctive diagnostic patterns, and lower urinary tract infection might be related to one of four particular diagnostic patterns. Each of these patterns would be treated in different ways; as the saying goes, "One disease, different treatments."

There is also the saying, "Different diseases, one treatment," reflecting the concept that many different diseases may be captured within one pattern. One contemporary text lists such diverse entities as nephritis (inflammation of the kidneys), dysfunctional uterine bleeding, pyelonephritis (inflammation of the kidney and its pelvis), and rheumatic heart disease under the diagnostic pattern of "disharmony between the heart and kidney."

Types of diagnostic patterns

- viscera and bowels
- *qi* and blood and fluids
- triple burner
- six evils
- channel patterns
- Five Phases
- six channels
- four levels
- eight principles
- three causes
- seven effects.

Treating patients

Once a diagnosis has been reached and, when relevant, a pattern has been identified, therapy begins. Treatment in Chinese medicine follows a fundamentally *allopathic* philosophy, that is, it addresses the disease with opposing measures. As described in *The Yellow Emperor's Inner Classic*, "Cold is treated with heat, heat is treated with cold, vacuity is treated by supplementation, and repletion is treated by drainage."

Within the realm of acupuncture, moxibustion (heating herbs on or near the skin), and herbal medicine, three fundamental principles of therapy are understood and applied: *treating disease at its root, eliminating evil influences and supporting right influences*, and *restoring the balance of yin and yang*. For instance, with our hypothetical wind-cold patient, the practitioner would seek to eliminate the cold evil and support the right *qi*. Where the symptoms reflect a more complex underlying pattern, the physician might attempt to treat the root of the patient's condition. Functional uterine bleeding due to a disharmony of the heart and kidney would be addressed primarily by harmonizing the heart and kidney; treating the root of the condition would adjust its symptoms at the uterine level.

The most common methods for treating health problems include acupuncture, moxibustion, cupping, bleeding, massage, *qi* cultivation (*qi gong*), herbal medicine, and diet.

Acupuncture and moxibustion can be used independently of each other but are so deeply wedded in Chinese medicine that the term for this therapy is *zhen jiu*, meaning "needle moxibustion," sometimes translated as "acumoxa therapy." Both techniques are used to provide a focused stimulus to points that lie along channel pathways, or to other appropriate sites. The basis of their close linkage lies in ancient origins of the methods and the fact that moxibustion appears to have been the first form of therapy applied to the channels and holes in order to treat problems on or within the body. We will address acupuncture and related practices in detail in Chapter 6.

Chapter 5

Diet, Foods, and Chinese Herbal Medicine

The cultivation of plants as food or medicine, and often food *and* medicine, has great antiquity and is closely associated with the rise of Chinese civilization itself through plant domestication, irrigation agriculture and massive state water works projects (see page 19).

Foods, nutrition, and diet

It is part of conventional wisdom in the West that many useful technologies were developed in ancient China, including animal domestication, plant cultivation and irrigation agriculture, to nourish large numbers of people. However, it is not as readily accepted that the Chinese civilization also developed thousands of effective medicines from plants and, to a lesser extent, from animal and mineral sources. *Just as plants are cultivated for nourishing foods, so they are for effective medicines.*

Four sacred grains

The agricultural properties of plants were known from early times in China. The *four sacred grains* (barley, millet, rice, and wheat) are represented in early Chinese pictographs that emphasize the above-ground, grain-producing, nourishing portions of these plants. That barley, millet, and wheat, also known to the West, were important is evidenced by northern Chinese cuisine, for example. However, the ability of *rice* to withstand periodic flooding and grow partially underwater (before the Chinese waterways were brought under control by state projects) gained it a prominent position throughout China. The ability of these grains to provide carbohydrates and calories to large, dense populations was an important factor in the rise of Chinese civilization.

However, these populations also require protein, as well as vitamins and minerals, the latter present in the unpolished husk of grains, such as brown rice and whole wheat, but removed by the milling processes that produce white rice and blanched wheat. We are familiar with the twentieth-century tragedy of famine in Asia, where children who were getting milled rice for calories suffered from protein deficiency (*kwashiorkor*), or vitamin B deficiencies such as *beri beri* and *pellagra*. Protein is harder to come by in the plant kingdom, except for the botanical species know as legumes (the large family and varieties of beans). In addition to the four sacred grains producing carbohydrate, another Chinese plant of agricultural importance was *soybean*.

Adding a fifth grain

Unlike the Chinese characters for the four sacred grains, the character for *soy* emphasizes the lower part of the pictograph, or the portion of the plant that is underground. Another characteristic of legumes, like soy, together with the protein they produce, is the ability of their roots to host nitrogen-fixing bacteria.

These legume plants allow specific bacteria to literally "take root" underground to pull nitrogen from the air and restore it to the soil—and so this remarkable plant replenishes soils that become exhausted through intensive growing of grains.

Counting for tastes and numbering the diet

Ancient Chinese wisdom calls for eating "the five cereals to nourish the vital *qi* of the five *Zhang* organs, together with the five fruits, the five meats, and the five vegetables" (*Suwen*). The center of the meal was grain, but a variety of foods should also be consumed. The five foods in each category also represent tastes. A satisfying meal should nourish the senses as well as the body. In the West, the foods with different tastes are taken in order, so that at the end of the meal, sweet taste buds still call for the stimulation of dessert. In Chinese and Asian cuisine the acrid, bitter, sweet, sour and salty tastes can all be mixed together in each dish, providing a fully satisfying sensory experience:

- sweet—rice
- sour (astringent)—sesame
- salty—soybeans
- bitter—wheat
- pungent (*ling shu*)—millet (broomcorn).

Missing from the Chinese diet is milk, and there is effectively no dairy industry, probably due to the high rate of lactose intolerance. However, it is arguable that humans are not designed to consume milk past infancy. In China, milk consumption is said to weaken the spleen, creating conditions of excess phlegm, such as asthma, fibroids, headaches and nasal congestion. The association of milk with allergies and these related symptoms is well noted in Western biomedicine.

Further, the ability to draw nitrogen from the atmosphere also allows leguminous plants to form the *amino acids* (nitrogen-based biochemicals) that in turn are the building blocks of *protein*. In the soybean, however, the nutritious proteins co-exist with other constituents that are virtually indigestible (but control predatory animals and insects as natural pesticides). These other substances include anti-tryptic factors which literally inhibit digestion (and in severe poisonings can cause the symptoms of cystic fibrosis). Somehow, through historical trial and error, the Chinese learned to prepare soy in various ways that eliminate the toxic poisons. For example, if soy is mixed with water, and then sea salt is added, (or soy is simply mixed with sea water), the calcium (chemical symbol Ca), magnesium (Mg) and other minerals in the sea salt combine with the soy proteins to form solids (technically a divalent cation protein precipitation, where minerals with two positive (++) chemical charges, like Ca++ and Mg++, combine with protein in water solution to form solids). These proteins precipitate from the water to form solids, leaving the toxic poisons behind in the water. When the water is squeezed out of the solid protein, as in the preparation of *tofu*, a nutritious food results. Another way to neutralize the poisons is to ferment the soy and add salts, creating the well-known soy sauce, which, when added to rice, forms a nutritious meal of carbohydrate and protein.

Diet as therapy

In addition to nourishment, diet can be used to prevent disease, promote longevity or help treat an existing condition. For treating disease, diet is usually employed as an adjunct to acupuncture and/or herbal medicine.

Dietary guidelines for disease are based upon the correspondences that apply in other areas of treatment. To soothe the liver *qi* and clear heat, the patient avoids liver-heating foods such as alcohol, coffee, cola, and red meat, so that these do not interfere with the treatments. The exclusion of certain foods is just as important as the prescription of others.

Digestion

Chinese medicine recognizes the role of a healthy digestive system in preventing and treating disease. The Zang-Fu organ system identified as the spleen and stomach correspond most closely to the functions of digestion and absorption in western medicine. The strength of the spleen and the stomach are considered critical to prevention of, and treatment or recovery from, essentially every condition, as they are responsible for taking in food and fluids, transforming them to *qi* and blood, and transporting them throughout the body.

In Chinese medicine, the *way* one eats is just as important for health as *what* one eats. Irregular eating times, eating in haste, and eating iced foods all weaken the function of spleen and stomach. Importantly, the state of the spleen–stomach functions are crucial to every condition in Chinese medicine. In Western medicine the state of digestion is considered only when it is the chief complaint, rather than being considered in all conditions.

Chinese diet therapy emphasizes that only foods of good quality, properly prepared, are health giving. As an ancient source, it does not directly address the problems of modern agricultural practices such as food processing and the use of antibiotics, herbicides, hormones, pesticides, irradiation, or genetic manipulation.

Likewise, ancient Chinese medicine does not consider terms such as nutrients or phytochemicals, although there is recognition that fresh foods (higher in nutrients) are preferable, and locally grown foods, being fresher, are considered better. Further, food is a source of *qi*. The vitality, or life force, remaining in the food is the main consideration.

Food or herbal medicine?

The properties in terms of which foods are considered are the same as those used for medicinal plants:

- five flavors
- four natures
- four directions
- channel propensity.

There is a fine line between foods and herbs, and they are often used together. Certainly, herbs as spices can be ingredients in preparation of foods for consumption. Plants contain biologically active constituents as a product of their evolution and growth in the terrestrial environment, where they compete for sustenance and against predation by animals, insects, fungi and bacteria. In fact, the antibacterial properties of many spices, allowing the preservation of meats and other foods, made them very valuable during the period of Portuguese, Spanish, Dutch, French and British exploration in Greater China, and were a prime motivator for establishing a European presence there. It is no accident that the Malaysian archipelago of Southeast Asia was long called the "Spice Islands" (see pages 153–154).

In general, strictly herbal preparations are stronger than food preparations and are meant to be used only for short periods of time.

The five flavors

As shown in Table 5.1, the five different tastes each have different actions in the body.

Table 5.1 The medicinal effects of the five flavors

Sour (including astringent)	Retains and arrests loss of fluids (for diarrhea, sweat), generates fluids, promotes proper digestion *Hawthorn berries (cardioactive), lemon, apricots, cherries, grapefruit (also sweet)*
Bitter	Drying and purging (for constipation, reflux, cough) *Bitter melon, dandelion greens*
Sweet	Tonifies and strengthens blood (for pain and spasms) *Chicken, eggs, fruits, mutton, root vegetables*
Pungent	Expels pathogens and promotes *qi* and blood flow. *Chilli, ginger, pepper, spring onions*
Salty	Softens and resolves masses (goiter) *Kelp, seaweed (iodine)*

Four natures, directions, and channel propensity

The *four natures* of foods correlate with the temperatures of cold, cool, warm and hot. The nature of the food is determined by its effect on the body. If it lowers a fever, it is considered cold. If it promotes blood circulation and warms the extremities, it is considered warm or hot.

Once food is digested it can have an impact on the *direction* of the flow of *qi*—*ascending, descending, floating,* and *sinking*:

- ascending—for diarrhea and organ prolapse

- descending—for belching and indigestion, hiccups, nausea, and vomiting

- floating (dispersing)—for common cold, promotes perspiration

- sinking—for constipation, high blood pressure, mania.

The *parts* of a plant food are also relevant. Flowers and leaves tend to move upward; fruits, roots and seeds tend to move downward—this is the sense of "direction."

The *propensity* determines the organ channel to which a food is likely to travel. Most foods go to at least two channels. For example, lemons, pears, and tangerines clear heat from the Lung channel to stop coughs. Tangerines also go to the Stomach channel to address loss of appetite and nausea.

The flavor, nature, direction and channel propensity of a food determine its medicinal value.

Seasonality

Just as time of day and the circumstances for food preparation and consumption are important, so are the four seasons. Beyond the fact that different foods are available in different seasons (sweet potatoes and root vegetables in winter; watermelon and salad greens in summer), in Chinese medicine the seasons have a direct effect on the body, which in turn indicates different foods to be appropriate:

- Spring: warming; more sweet than sour foods, to nourish spleen *qi* when liver *qi* is strong.

- Summer: hot; digestion slows; light foods to clear heat and generate fluids; more fruits and vegetables, less meat.

- Autumn: cooling; avoid extremes of hot or cold; Yang-Qi diminishing (energy), yin-qi (substance) growing; foods moderate in nature.

- Winter: cold; tonify and rebalance; yang-qi deficient, yin-qi in excess; beef, mutton, nourishing and invigorating diet.

Living inside controlled environments works against the natural effects of the seasonal cycle. Excessive indoor cooling when temperatures should normally be hot in summer, and dry heating when temperatures should be cold in winter, require modifications: add some warming foods to the light summer diet of fruits and vegetables; tonify with moistening foods in winter.

Geographic location also influences seasonal climate. In hot, humid climates, "damp" disorders will be worse in later summer, while in hot, dry, desert climates, "dry" disorders may worsen in autumn.

The aging process mirrors the seasons. In children, internal damp syndromes frequently lead to nasal congestion and running, asthma and ear infections. Cold and moist foods such as dairy products aggravate damp conditions and should be avoided for children. The elderly have weakening digestive functions and should have small, frequent meals, well-cooked and easily digestible soups and stews.

In pregnant women, fluids collect in certain channels, leaving others relatively dry, so drying foods such as spices and wines should be avoided.

Emotional states also have an effect on digestion. Stress hinders proper function of spleen and stomach and requires a diet that tonifies the spleen and is easy to digest. Anger and disappointment require a diet that soothes the liver *qi*.

Preparation

Healthy food preparation begins with selection based upon cleanliness, color intensity, texture, and fragrance. A key principle is making food that is easy to digest while retaining its nourishing value and vitality; this includes cutting foods into proper shapes and sizes and using appropriate cooking methods and condiments. Classic Chinese cuisine accomplishes healthy cooking by quickly heating small pieces of food, making them easy to digest and preserving nutritional value by not overheating or overcooking. Steaming, braising, stir-frying, stewing, roasting, and quick boiling are common methods, used as suited to particular foods. Frequently added condiments include cilantro, chilli, garlic, ginger, mustard, pepper, and spring onion.

A medicinal diet can be dispensed in the form of teas, decoctions, juices, wines, gruels (with rice and millet), soups, pancakes, candied fruits, and other forms.

The healthful properties of foods are maintained or enhanced through proper cultivation, selection, preparation, consumption and digestion. Each step in this process "from field to table," to spleen–stomach, is given attention in Chinese medicine. The properties of foods are similar to those ascribed to medicinal plants and other healthful influences on *qi*, blood, and body.

Medicinal plants

Since the legendary emperor Shen Nong first tasted herbs and guided the Chinese people in their classification, the use of medicinal plants, or herbal medicine, has been an integral part of Chinese culture and medical practice. The traditional Chinese *materia medica* includes minerals and animal products as well as herbs. There are nearly 5800 substances recorded in the *Encyclopedia of Traditional Chinese Medicinal Substances* (*Zhong Yao Da Ci Dian*) published in 1977 by the Jiangsu College of New Medicine. This publication is a later entry in a long line of definitive discussions of *materia medica* that have been produced in China over the millennia. The earliest known work, *The Divine Husbandman's Classic of the Materia Medica*, was reconstructed by Tao Hong Jing (452–536 CE).

Assimilation of new herbs into the ancient pharmacopeia

The ancient pharmacopeia continues to grow with assimilation of herbs from global geographic regions. For example, when Chinese laborers were employed by the Union Pacific Railroad for the construction of the western half of the U.S. transcontinental railroad completed in 1869, they encountered North American herbs (many already known as Native American remedies) and quickly expanded the 3000-year-old Chinese pharmacopeia to incorporate these new discoveries. In this way the potent American ginseng was added alongside Siberian ginseng and Chinese ginseng. The properties of American ginseng, already highly valued by Native Americans, had quickly become known to the European settlers, and it became an important economic product, driving many literally into the mountains of Appalachia to collect it. The desire for ginseng stimulated exploration and eventually westward expansion. The famous early American frontier hero, Daniel Boone (America's version of a semi-mythical figure, such as personages we have seen in Chinese medical tradition), began by exploring the early western frontier of the Appalachians as a "sanger," gathering the valuable herb in the hills and hollows where it could be found (what today would be called "wildcrafting").

This text classified upper-, middle-, and lower-grade herbs, and discussed the tastes, temperatures, toxicities, and medicinal properties of 364 substances.

Today medicinal substances are categorized systematically as expansions of the methods of therapy. There are prescribing rules that take into account the compatibility or incompatibility of various substances, traditional pairings of substances, and combinations that address specific symptoms.

Categories of herbal medicines in the Chinese materia medica

- blood-rectifying
- ejecting
- exterior-resolving
- external use
- food-dispersing
- heat-clearing
- interior-warming
- liver-calming, wind-extinguishing
- orifice-opening
- phlegm-transforming, cough-suppressing, panting-calming
- precipitant
- *qi*-rectifying
- securing and astringing
- spirit-quieting
- supplementing
- water-disinhibiting, dampness-percolating
- wind-dispelling
- worm-expelling.

Not all herbal prescriptions are based on these theoretical diagnostic principles; many are selected on the basis of specific symptoms, possibly derived from the practical experience of the general population. Even today, despite the traditional diagnostic theory and pattern diagnosis that drives most herbal prescriptions in China, there are also extensive compilations of herbal formulas based on symptoms.

In the case of someone who has encountered a wind-cold evil or who, in the pattern identification system described in the *Treatise on Cold Damage*, would be said to have a *tai yang* stage pattern, a decoction of the herb ephedra (*ma huang tang*) would be an appropriate choice, particularly if the patient had a slight cough as well. The constituents and dosage of the formula are nine grams of ephedra, six grams of cinnamon twig (*gui zhi*), nine grams of apricot kernel (*xing ren*), and three grams of licorice (*gan cao*). These ingredients are boiled in water to make a concentrated tea or decoction, which the patient drinks warm in successive doses. This induces sweating, a sign that the *qi* of the surface of the body is free to move and throw off the evil. Once sweating begins, the patient stops drinking the decoction.

Ingredients in a traditional formula are identified as the *ruler, minister, adjutant,* and *emissary,* analogous to the governmental roles in ancient Chinese social organization (see page 18). The *ruler* sets the therapeutic direction of the formula. In this case, the ruler of the formula is ephedra, which is acrid and warm; it promotes sweating, dispels cold, and resolves the surface. Cinnamon twig is the *minister*, working to assist the ruler in carrying out its objectives; in addition, cinnamon itself is said to warm the body. Apricot kernel is the *adjutant*, and so addresses the possible involvement of the lung and moderates the acrid flavor of the two other substances. Finally, licorice is the *emissary*, serving both to render the action of the other herbs harmonious and to distribute them through the body.

The foregoing is a brief, simple example of Chinese herbal therapy, which can be quite complex and is capable of addressing an even broader range of conditions than acupuncture. In terms of complexity and the diagnostic acumen required of the practitioner, it resembles the Western practice of *internal medicine*. Herbal therapy encompasses the external applications of herbs as well as internal doses taken in the form of powder, pills, pastes, or tinctures, as well as the traditional water decoction.

Chinese *foods and herbs* have been used for medicinal purposes since antiquity. *The Yellow Emperor's Inner Classic* discusses therapeutic application of the *Five Phase Theory* to foods, and today it is not unusual to see a classroom kitchen in a college of Chinese medicine. In larger Chinese cities, special restaurants prepare meals for specific medicinal purposes.

The practices of this field are deeply rooted in the cultural practices of China and the culture's beliefs concerning diet. Many of the foods that are used in medical therapy also are routinely prepared by families when seasons change, when illness strikes, to strengthen a woman after birth, to cause milk to fill the breasts of a new mother, or to nourish the elderly in their declining years.

Health benefits of Chinese medicinal plants

The study of Chinese plants, foods and herbal medicine has yielded a rich store of high-quality information, much of which has been translated into English. It primarily covers two areas: (1) the pharmaceutical properties of substances, and (2) their clinical effectiveness. Scientists in China, Japan, and, more recently, the United States and Europe have found it fairly easy to conduct studies to identify and isolate apparently active compounds.

A famous case in point is that of the very first herb listed in the Chinese *materia medica*: *herba ephedra*, known botanically as *Ephedra sinica*, and in Chinese as *ma huang*. Ephedra is recorded in *The Divine Husbandman's Classic of the Materia Medica*. Its chief active component, ephedrine, was isolated in 1887 in Japan, but remained largely unexplored for 35 years. Then Carl F. Schmidt from the University of Pennsylvania and K. K. Chen began to study its pharmacological effects at the Peking Union Medical College, where the department of pharmacology was beginning a systematic exploration of the Chinese *materia medica*.

These investigations revealed that ephedrine produced effects similar to epinephrine (also known as adrenaline), such as increasing blood pressure, constricting blood vessels, and dilating the bronchial tubes. Epinephrine is commonly administered by injection for various conditions. Ephedrine has distinct advantages over epinephrine: it can be administered orally, has a longer duration of action, and is less toxic. It has proved useful in managing bronchial asthma and hay fever, and in supporting a patient's vital signs during spinal anesthesia. When ephedrine was later synthesized, it was used in a number of pharmaceuticals, including such over-the-counter products as Sudafed and Actifed.

Ephedra represents an early and impressive example of the benefits of research into Chinese herbs. Other examples of single herbs that have proven useful in clinical experiments include *herba artemisiae* (*yin chen hao*) for hepatitis and malaria, and *caulis mu tong* (*mu tong*) for urinary tract infections.

With more than 5000 substances known in traditional Chinese medicine, the scope of study is quite large, even more so because many of these substances are combined in formulas and administered by means of a complex system of pattern identification and diagnosis. However, it is possible to design effective studies, as demonstrated in a project conducted by Alan Bensoussan under the auspices of the Research Unit for Complementary Medicine, University of Western Sydney, Macarthur, in Australia. Other studies in Chinese herbal medicine taking place in Asia, Europe, North America, and Australia are revealing tremendous potential for their use in modern health care (see Chapters 16 and 17).

See Appendix I for details of the important Chinese medicinal plants (foods and herbal remedies) that are used today for their health benefits by tens of millions of people worldwide, and which are available to you now as safe and effective treatments for many common conditions.

Chapter 6

Acupuncture and Moxibustion

The therapeutic goal of acupuncture is to regulate *qi*. When *qi* and blood flow freely through the body, the person is in a state of health. When the flow of *qi* is interrupted by some cause—such as an evil, a disturbed mental state, or a trauma—illness results and pain can occur. Pain is directly linked to an injury or to interruption of the flow of *qi*. Acupuncture is employed to remove the obstruction and restore the flow. Needling may be used to remove the evil, to direct *qi* to places where it is insufficient, or to cause *qi* to flow where it previously had been blocked.

The "Spiritual Axis" of *The Yellow Emperor's Inner Classic* described *nine needles* for use in acupuncture. With the exception of one that appears to have had a specifically surgical application, these needle types are still in use today, in either original or adapted form. Modern acupuncture also includes other tools and methods that have been added over the centuries.

The most common acupuncture tool is the filiform, or fine, needle, which can vary significantly in terms of structure, diameter, and length. A typical acupuncture needle has a body or shaft that is one inch long and a handle of approximately the same length. The distinctive part of an acupuncture needle is its tip, which is rounded and moderately sharp, much like the tip of a pine needle. Solid and gently tapered, the acupuncture needle does not have the cutting edge of a hollow-point hypodermic needle. Its diameter typically is 0.25 mm (0.01 inch) or less.

Sticking to it

Once the site for insertion has been determined, the needle is inserted rapidly through the skin and then adjusted to an appropriate depth. A twelfth-century CE text, *Ode of the Subtleties of Flow*, states, "Insert the needle with noble speed, then proceed [to the appropriate depth] slowly; withdraw the needle with noble slowness, as haste will cause injury." Although a substantial number of considerations affect the angle and depth of insertion, methods of manipulation, and length of retention, the following description outlines a basic procedure.

The essential aim is to *obtain qi* at the needling site, and the acupuncturist seeks either an objective or a subjective indication that the *qi* has arrived. The practitioner can sense *qi* through his or her hands as the needle is manipulated, or can determine its presence through observation of its effects and/or reports from the patient. The practitioner often feels the arrival of *qi* as a gentle grasping of the needle at the site, like a fish on the end of a line. The patient may sense the arrival of *qi* as itching, numbness, soreness, a swollen feeling, a local temperature change, or a distinct "electrical" sensation. Acupuncture points in different areas of the body respond differently, and these variations in response can be an important diagnostic indicator. It is not unusual for a clinician to retain a needle in an acupuncture point where the *qi* has not arrived, until the characteristic sensation eventually occurs.

Once *qi* has been obtained, the clinician may choose to manipulate the needle to achieve a desired therapeutic effect. Methods range from simply putting the needle in place and leaving it there, to engaging in complex manipulations that involve slow or rapid insertion of the needle to greater or more shallow depths. These techniques may create a distinctive sensation along the channel pathway. The needle may be withdrawn promptly after *qi* arrives, or a short, fine needle (known as an intradermal) may be retained in the site for several days. In all instances, the goal of the clinician is to influence the movement of *qi*.

One simple style of needle manipulation involves adjusting the direction of the needle to supplement or drain the *qi* at the particular channel point. If the acupuncture point is visualized as a hole where the channel *qi* can be touched and moved, this operation can either cause the *qi* to become secure and increase in the channel (supplementing), or cause the *qi* to spill out (draining).

For a patient who is experiencing the symptoms of wind cold, an acupuncturist might choose to needle a number of acupuncture points including: *Wind Pool* (*Feng Chi GB 20*), located on the back of the neck below the occipital bone; *Union Valley* (*He Gu LI 4*), located in the fleshy area between the base of the thumb and forefinger; and *Broken Sequence* (*Lie Que LU 7*), on the forearm. These particular points could all be treated with a draining method since, in this case, the channels are replete with the influences of the external evils of wind and cold. Wind Pool, as its name indicates, is often used to drain wind from the surface of the body, relieving headache and neck pain. Union Valley is an important acupuncture point that is used to influence the upper part of the body and to control pain. In this case, the point is used because of its ability to redirect wind, resolve the exterior, and to treat headache and sore throat. Broken Sequence is said to dispel cold and to diffuse the lung. It affects the channels and can be used to treat sore throat and headache.

Another way to choose acupuncture points is based on their associations with the Five Phases (see Chapter 3). Each of the phases corresponds to an organ, as outlined in the box on the following page.

Each phase is also related to a number of other categories, including taste, smell, climate, and time of day. If the patient displayed signs of vacuity of the Water phase, a choice of points could be made from the transport points along the kidney channel associated with Water, in order to supplement the Water phase.

The Five Phase correspondences

- Wood to Liver
- Fire to Heart
- Earth to Spleen
- Metal to Lungs
- Water to Kidney.

Points also may be chosen on the basis of the actual anatomic *trajectory of the channel* upon which they lie on the body. Union Valley is considered an important point for the head and face because the pathway of the large intestine channel, on which it lies, traverses that area of the body. Similarly, points on the lower extremity that lie on the urinary bladder channel, which traverses the entire back, are frequently used for back pain.

Finally, the practitioner often selects acupuncture points entirely on the basis of their *sensitivity to palpation*, or on the basis of a variation in texture that the practitioner can perceive. Often, a number of acupuncture points in a specific area may be assessed to determine which would be most suitable for needling. In some cases, points that do not lie on specific channels, or form part of the collection of recognized extra points, may be identified by their tenderness. These points are known as *ah shi*, or "ouch, that's it," points, and are an important part of clinical acupuncture's traditional history and contemporary practice.

With so many acupuncture points to choose from and so many methods for choosing them, it is not surprising that many clinicians focus on a few specific methods, or a particular collection of points, so that they can develop expertise in the application of those key treatments.

Moxibustion (*jiu fa*)

Moxibustion refers to the burning of dried and powdered leaves of *Artemesia vulgaris* (*ai ye*) or wormwood on or near the skin in order to affect the movement of *qi* in the channel. *A. vulgaris* is said to be acrid and bitter and, when used as moxa, to have the ability to warm and enter channels. References to moxa appear in very early materials, such as the texts recovered from excavated tombs at Ma Wang Dui, which date to 168 BCE.

Moxibustion can be applied to the body in many ways: *directly, indirectly, by pole moxa,* and *by the warm needle method.*

Direct moxa involves burning a small amount of moxa, about the size of a grain of rice, directly on the skin. Depending on the desired effect, larger or smaller pieces of moxa may be used, and the moxa fluff can either be allowed to burn all the way to the skin, causing a blister or a scar, or it can be removed before it has reached the skin. These techniques are used to stimulate acupuncture points where the action of moxibustion is traditionally indicated, or where warming the point seems to be the most appropriate response.

Indirect moxibustion involves the insertion of a substance between the moxa fluff and the patient's skin. This gives the practitioner greater control over the degree of heat applied to the patient's body and offers the patient increased protection from burning, allowing moxa treatments in such delicate areas as the face and back. Popular substances placed between moxa and the skin include ginger slices, garlic slices, and salt. The substance is often chosen because it has medicinal properties of its own that combine well with the properties of moxa. For instance, ginger might be selected in cases where vacuity cold is present, while garlic is considered useful for treating hot and toxic conditions.

During *pole moxa*, a cigar-shaped roll of moxa wrapped in paper is used to warm the acupuncture points gently without touching the skin. This is a very safe method of moxibustion that can be taught to patients for self-application.

The *warm needle method* is accomplished by first inserting an acupuncture needle into the point and then placing moxa fluff on its handle. After the moxa is ignited, it burns gradually, imparting a sensation of gentle warmth to the acupuncture point and channel. This method is especially useful for people with arthritic joint pain.

Together, acupuncture and moxibustion are used to address a wide range of conditions and symptoms. Based on the basic concept that all disease ultimately involves disruption of the flow of *qi*, and that acupuncture and moxibustion regulate the movement of *qi*, there is no disease that could not benefit from these methods.

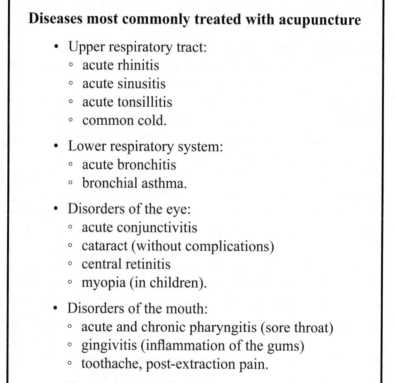

Diseases most commonly treated with acupuncture

- Upper respiratory tract:
  - acute rhinitis
  - acute sinusitis
  - acute tonsillitis
  - common cold.

- Lower respiratory system:
  - acute bronchitis
  - bronchial asthma.

- Disorders of the eye:
  - acute conjunctivitis
  - cataract (without complications)
  - central retinitis
  - myopia (in children).

- Disorders of the mouth:
  - acute and chronic pharyngitis (sore throat)
  - gingivitis (inflammation of the gums)
  - toothache, post-extraction pain.

- Gastrointestinal disorders:
  - acute bacillary dysentery
  - acute and chronic colitis
  - acute and chronic gastritis
  - acute duodenal ulcer (without complications)
  - chronic duodenal ulcer (used for pain relief)

- ○ constipation
- ○ diarrhea
- ○ gastric hyperacidity
- ○ gastroptosis (downward displacement of stomach)
- ○ hiccups
- ○ spasms of esophagus and cardia (junction of esophagus and stomach)
- ○ paralytic ileus (intestinal obstruction).

- • Neurological and musculoskeletal disorders:
  - ○ cervicobrachial syndrome (disease of neck and arm)
  - ○ facial palsy (early stage, i.e., within three to six months of onset)
  - ○ frozen shoulder, tennis elbow
  - ○ headache and migraine
  - ○ intercostal neuralgia (pain between the ribs)
  - ○ low back pain
  - ○ Meniére's disease (auditory vertigo)
  - ○ neurogenic bladder dysfunction
  - ○ nocturnal enuresis (involuntary urination)
  - ○ osteoarthritis
  - ○ pareses (paralysis) following a stroke
  - ○ peripheral neuropathies (nerve disorders)
  - ○ sciatica
  - ○ sequelae (complications) of poliomyelitis (early stage, i.e., within six months of onset)
  - ○ trigeminal neuralgia (shooting pains in the face).

Auricular acupuncture

The stimulation of acupoints on the external ear is a style of traditional acupuncture that integrates both Asian and Western approaches to health care. While the earliest clinical records of ear acupuncture points can be traced back to ancient Chinese texts written 2000 years ago, the style in which auricular acupuncture is currently practiced in modern China and throughout the rest of the world originated with the work of a French physician in 1957.

Instead of the traditional array of acupuncture points on the ear that had been used by ancient Chinese doctors, Dr. Paul Nogier of Lyons, France, proposed that the auricle can be perceived as an inverted fetus. Medical conditions associated with the head and face are treated by ear reflex points on the lower regions of the auricle, dysfunctions of the neck and upper back by points found on middle regions of the auricle, and pain or pathology in the lower back, leg, and foot by points on the highest regions of the external ear. Nogier's original report of an inverted, somatotopic pattern on the external ear was first presented at a scientific meeting in France, then distributed internationally by a German publication, next translated into Japanese, and finally printed in China. By 1958, the Nanjing Army Ear Acupuncture Research Team had conducted a clinical survey of 2000 patients who had been successfully treated with auricular acupuncture alone.

Many Western scientists remain skeptical of the concept that the organization of auricular acupoints exhibits a somatotopic arrangement. However, human brain imaging studies demonstrate greater responses in the area of the brain's somatic cortex that corresponds to the hand, when the hand area of the auricle is activated by acupoint stimulation.

Classical acupuncture theory attributes health and disease to the blockage of energy flow along acupuncture meridians (invisible lines of force extending over the surface of the body). Only the yang acupuncture meridians directly connect to the acupuncture points on the external ear. As with body acupuncture, the purported ability of auricular acupoints to heal is attributed to the increased flow of *qi* energetic forces throughout the body. Nogier was knowledgeable about the Chinese energetic perspective of the human body, but he also emphasized ontogenetic and neurophysiological connections between auricular reflex points and the central nervous system in order to explain the somatotopic relations between auricular regions and body pathology.

In his subsequent writings, Nogier proposed that there are three different territories on the external ear which are related to different types of neural innervation and three different types of embryological tissue. These three territories of the auricle can be viewed as three concentric rings:

- The *embryologically-based endodermal organs* are found *at the central concha of the ear*.

- The *mesodermal tissue that becomes the somatic musculature* is represented *on the middle ridges of the auricle*.

- The *ectodermal skin and nervous system tissue* are represented *on the outer ridges of the ear*.

The central concha of the ear is actually innervated by the vagus nerve and serves as the region for autonomic regulation of visceral pain and pathology associated with internal organs. The surrounding antihelix and antitragus ridges of the ear are innervated by the somatic trigeminal cranial nerve, and are used to treat myofascial pain that contributes to headaches, backaches, and body aches in the limbs. The outer rim of the auricle represents central nervous system pathways that affect neuropathic pain, such as peripheral neuropathies and trigeminal neuralgia. The ear lobe, at the bottom of the auricle, corresponds to the brain, whereas the outer helix tail of the auricle represents the spinal cord and spinal nerves.

Auricular master points

Auricular acupuncture treatments are by means of:

1. electrical stimulation of low electrical resistance acupoints on the ear

2. insertion of half inch needles into ear points based upon established treatment protocols

3. application of pressure by small "acubeads" taped to the ear.

The first set of ear acupoints considered for stimulation are referred to as "master points" and "supportive points." These auricular points do not correspond to one specific body organ, but affect many different medical conditions.

The first two master points, *Point Zero* and *Shen Men*, are utilized in most auriculotherapy treatment plans for the alleviation of several health disorders. *Point Zero* was first described by Nogier and is found in a notch on the helix root as it rises from the concha ridge. Point Zero functions as a homeostatic balancing point which leads to normalizing of dysfunctional conditions. The *Shen Men* point is the most frequently utilized ear point found in most Chinese treatment protocols, serving to alleviate stress, pain, tension, anxiety, depression, and substance abuse disorders. The English translation of the name of this ear acupuncture point is "Spirit Gate," suggesting that activation of this auricular point connects an individual to their *spiritual essence*, enhancing the vital forces of life and one's general well-being. The physical location of Shen Men is toward the tip of the triangular fossa. Detection of auricular points by an electrodermal point finder typically reveals that Point Zero and Shen Men are electrically reactive in most medical patients.

Two master points used in many neurological conditions and pain disorders are the *Autonomic Sympathetic point*, the name of which refers to its use in regulating the autonomic nervous system, and the *Thalamus* or *Subcortex point*, representing a brain region that serves as a higher brain center for the control of pain. The Autonomic Sympathetic point is found on the underside of the internal helix, where it meets the antihelix inferior crus. The Thalamus point is found on the base of the concha wall, behind the antitragus.

The *Endocrine point* is a nearby region of the intertragic notch which represents the pituitary gland, the master control gland for all other endocrine glands. Stimulation of this auricular point affects circulating hormones, such as cortisol and endorphins, whose levels are frequently altered during many conditions associated with pain and stress.

At the center of the ear lobe, vertically below Point Zero, is the *Master Sensorial point*, used to alleviate any disturbing somatic sensations.

Located central to this point on the ear lobe is the *Master Cerebral point*, also referred to as the *neurasthenia* or "worry point." Its stimulation is utilized to contain pathological obsessions, unwarranted worry and generalized anxiety.

Musculoskeletal auricular points

In his original text, *The Treatise of Auriculotherapy*, Nogier focused on auricular representation of the musculoskeletal body because practitioners new to auriculotherapy could confirm for themselves that specific regions of electrical conductivity and tenderness on the external ear corresponded to specific areas of the body where the patient felt myofascial discomfort. The cervical vertebrae are represented on the concha side of the antihelix tail, the thoracic vertebrae are represented on the central side of the antihelix body, and the lumbo-sacral vertebrae are represented on the inferior crus of the antihelix. The posterior groove behind each level of the antihelix is also stimulated to effectively reduce pain from muscle spasms.

The occiput is appropriately represented on the antitragus region adjacent to the lowest portion of the antihelix tail, which corresponds to the upper cervical spine. Toward the middle of the antitragus is found the auricular microsystem point for the temples, and toward the base of the antitragus, near the intertragic notch, is the Forehead point. The most reactive of these antitragus auricular points is utilized to treat both tension headaches and migraines.

At the junction of the upper regions of the ear lobe and the lower sections of the scaphoid fossa is found the TMJ (temporomandibular joint) point that is used for the relief of tight and tense muscles of the lower and upper jaw.

In Chinese auricular charts, the hip, knee, ankle and foot are represented in an upside-down arrangement on the superior crus of the antihelix. The somatotopic presentation of these same leg points in the European system is also found in an inverted orientation, but located in the triangular fossa.

As with vertebral points, stimulation of the posterior side of the triangular fossa and the superior crus serves to enhance the relief of myofascial pain in the legs or feet.

There is no discrepancy between European and Chinese ear charts which indicate auricular representation of the upper extremities. Treatment of shoulder problems is achieved by stimulation of a point in the scaphoid fossa peripheral to Point Zero. The Shoulder point is logically located next to the junction of auricular representation of the cervical spine and the thoracic spine. Since the somatotopic system on the ear is in an inverted orientation, the Elbow point is found in the region of the scaphoid fossa above the Shoulder point, and as one ascends higher in the scaphoid fossa, one arrives at the Wrist point, above which are several points for the fingers. Both the front and the back side of the ear are stimulated to relieve tennis elbow, carpal tunnel syndrome, and arthritic pain in the fingers (Oleson 1996).

Visceral disorders

Points for visceral organs derived from endodermal embryological tissue are found in the central valley of the auricle, the concha. It is intriguing to know that the only location on the body where the autonomic vagus nerve reaches the superficial skin is in the region of the concha floor. Near the opening to the actual auditory canal is the opening to the digestive system, the mouth. Extending peripherally from the auditory canal is the Esophagus point, which leads to the Stomach point found on the concha ridge. Stimulation of the auricular Stomach point in animals reduces neuronal firing rates in the feeding center of the hypothalamus, and neuronal discharges in the satiety center of the hypothalamus are increased by auricular stimulation. On the superior concha is found auricular representation of the small intestines and the large intestines. Stimulation of these points relieves physiological dysfunctions in each organ, such as nausea, diarrhea or constipation; or it may alter the energetic function of the corresponding acupuncture meridian named for that organ. Several studies have shown that stimulation of ear reflex points for the stomach can alter physiological patterns in the nervous connections between the gastro-intestinal tract and the hypothalamus in the brain.

The *Five Element Theory* suggests that the five yin organs affect problems of energetic constitution, as well as the known physiological functions of those organs:

- The kidney is energetically related to neurological and hearing disorders as well as physiological urinary dysfunctions.

- The liver can energetically affect tendon and ligament sprains, as well as hepatitis.

- The spleen can energetically alleviate muscle spasms, as well as affect lymphatic disorders.

- The lung is energetically used to treat skin disorders and drug detoxification, as well as respiratory problems.

- The heart is energetically utilized for mental calming, as well as cardiovascular irregularities.

(Oleson 2001, pp.221–233)

The auricular point for the heart is found at the very center of the Inferior Concha, in the deepest region of the concha floor, but Nogier has shown an additional heart point on the antihelix area where the chest is represented. Coronary heart disease would be treated in both locations.

Nervous system tissue is derived from ectodermal tissues that are represented on the lower regions of the external ear. The ear lobe and the antitragus above it represent the face and head, but also the brain inside the head. At the intertragic notch there is represented the anterior cingulate gyrus, an area of the limbic system which has been found to be very active in pain patients and which can be suppressed by body acupuncture stimulation. Stimulation of the cingulate gyrus ear point is effective in relieving chronic pain in human patients. The other important auricular points for pain relief are the thalamus point and the brain point, both found on the concha wall behind the antitragus.

It may seem almost "too good to be true" that such a simple procedure can effectively alleviate pain and disorders in so many different parts of the body. Nonetheless, practitioners of this approach have repeatedly observed that specific areas of the auricle are more sensitive to pressure and more electrically active, in a predictable pattern that conforms to the inverted fetus perspective that Nogier first discovered in the 1950s. Activation of these auricular points with needle insertion, transcutaneous electrical stimulation, or application of pressure pellets, has been shown to alleviate physical symptoms in the corresponding part of the body.

The use of auricular acupuncture has increased in China, Europe, and the United States as a result of repeated clinical experience of the effectiveness of this technique. That neurological reflexes could connect distant regions of the body to somatotopic microsystems on the ear suggests a kind of neuronal organization that has apparently been discovered outside the current boundaries of current Western medical science and practice.

Chapter 7

Manual Methods and Chinese Massage

There are a number of techniques within classic Chinese medical practice, and derived from Chinese medical practice, that *make use of the knowledge of vital energy and acupuncture points and meridians* but *without using needles* to influence them. These may be particularly appealing to individuals who are "needle phobic," or in situations where sterile needles are not available.

Tui na: manual acupuncture point stimulation (Chinese massage)

Tui na (literally "pushing and pulling") is a system of massage, manual acupuncture point stimulation, and manipulation that is vast enough to warrant a modality of its own. These methods have been practiced at least as long as moxibustion, if not longer, but the first formal massage training class was not held until 1956 in Shanghai. Today, this field of study can be a minor component of a traditional medical education, or a subject for extensive clinical specialization.

A distinctive aspect of *tui na* is the extensive training necessary for clinical practice. The practitioner's hands are taught to accomplish focused and forceful movements that can be applied to various areas of the body. Techniques such as pushing, rolling, kneading, rubbing, and grasping are repeated until they become second nature. Students practice on a small bag of rice until their hands develop the necessary strength and dexterity.

Tui na is often applied to highly localized areas of the body, and the techniques can be quite forceful and intense. Conditions routinely treated with *tui na* include *orthopedic and neurological conditions, asthma, dysmenorrhea (menstrual pain),* and *chronic gastritis.*

Tui na is used as an adjunct to acupuncture treatment to increase the range of motion of a joint, or instead of acupuncture if needles are uncomfortable or inappropriate, as, for example, when the patient is very young or old, or is "needle phobic."

As with all aspects of Chinese medicine, there are many regional styles and distinctive family lineages of practice. The formal curriculum available in Chinese programs is extensive, but still does not cover all the possibilities.

Acupressure and jin shin do

Acupressure is the application of the fingers to acupuncture points on the body, or "acupuncture without needles." It is based on the meridian or channel system, which informs other Chinese medical practices. According to this system, there are 12 major channels through which vital energy, or *qi*, flows. Although most of the channels are named for specific organs, they do not necessarily correspond to the anatomical body part, but rather are more functional in nature. Interruptions in the flow of *qi* cause functional aberrations associated with that particular channel. These interruptions can be released by specific application of needles or fingers.

Jin shin do, or the "way of the compassionate spirit," was developed by psychotherapist Iona Teeguarden. It is a form of acupressure in which the fingers are used to apply deep pressure to hypersensitive acupuncture points. *Jin shin do* represents a synthesis of Daoist philosophy, psychology, breathing, and acupressure techniques. According to this philosophy, the body is linked to the mind and spirit, and tender points found in the body can represent expressions of emotional trauma or locked memories (somato-emotional component).

The theory of *jin shin do* states that various stimuli cause energy to accumulate in acupuncture points. Repeated stress, in turn, causes a layering of tension at the point, known as *armoring*. The most painful point is termed the *local point* as a frame of reference. Other related tender points are referred to as *distal points*. Deep pressure applied to a point ultimately causes a release, and the tension dissipates. The overall effect is to reestablish flow in the channel and balance body energy. The context of the *jin shin do* treatment is as much psychological as physical and reiterates the importance of the body–mind–spirit philosophy of this treatment form.

During the treatment session the practitioner identifies a local point and "asks permission," nonverbally, to treat it. One finger is placed on the local point, and another finger is applied to a distal point. Gradually increasing pressure is applied to the local point. After one or two minutes the practitioner feels the muscle relaxing, followed by a pulsation (practitioners of cranio-sacral therapy refer to this phenomenon as the "therapeutic pulse"). When the pulsing stops, the patient usually reports decreased sensitivity at the point, indicating successful treatment. Myofascial (muscle-connective tissue) releases are sometimes accompanied by emotional releases as painful memories rise to consciousness.

Reflexology

In the Chinese meridian system of the body, all the major meridians or channels are represented in the hands and feet. Acupuncture is usually not done on the soles of the feet because of their sensitivity. (The feet, hands and face are very dense in sensory nerves.) Therefore, a system of foot massage was developed in China.

William H. Fitzgerald (1872–1942), who called it "zone therapy," introduced this Chinese system to the West in 1913. Now called *reflexology*, the technique involves deep pressure applied by the thumbs and fingers of the practitioner to various points on the patient's hands and feet. The feet receive the most attention in this method, with various identified points corresponding to the energy channels of the body and also to specific organs and systems.

When treatment is given, areas of tenderness or skin texture changes are identified and pressure is applied. This procedure has the effect of opening the corresponding channel, allowing body energy to flow unimpeded through the entirety of the channel and to the affected organs. When all relevant points have been successfully treated, the energy system is flowing and balanced.

Stimulation of these reflex areas helps the body to correct, strengthen, and reinforce itself by returning to a state of homeostasis. In Asian countries, some reflexologists also use electrical or mechanical devices. However, these approaches are discouraged in Europe and North America.

In the zone

Fitzgerald's studies found that pressure applied to various locations on the body also deadened sensation in definite areas and relieved pain. These findings led him to develop *zone therapy*. In the early years, Fitzgerald worked mainly on the hands. Later, the feet became very popular as a site for treatment. In his book on zone therapy (1917), Fitzgerald described working on the palmar surface of the hand for any pains in the back of the body, and working on the dorsal aspect of the hands and fingers for any problems on the anterior (front) part of the body.

Joe Shelby Riley, MD, was taught zone therapy by Dr. Fitzgerald. He developed and refined the techniques and created detailed diagrams and drawings of the reflex points located on the feet (Riley 1924).

As noted above, reflexology is based on the premise that there are zones and reflexes in different parts of the body that correspond to all parts, glands, and organs. Manipulating specific reflexes relieves stress, activating a parasympathetic nerve response that enables release through a physiological change in the body. With stress removed and circulation enhanced, the body is able to return to a state of homeostasis.

Conventional zone theory (CZT) is the foundation of hand and foot reflexology. *Zones* represent a system for organizing relations among various parts, glands, and organs of the body, and the nervous reflexes. There are ten equal, longitudinal or vertical zones running the length of the body, from the tips of the toes and fingers to the top of the head. From the dividing center line of the body, there are five zones on the right side, and five zones on the left side. These zones are numbered 1 to 5 from the medial side (inside) to the lateral side (outside). Each finger and toe falls into one of the five zones; for example, the left thumb is in the same zone as the left big toe: zone 1. Reflexology zones, as developed in this system, are not the same as acupuncture or acupressure meridians.

The reflexes are considered to pass all the way through the body, within the same zones. The same reflex, for example, can be found on the front and also on the back of the body, and on both surfaces of the hand or foot. Pressure applied to any part of a zone affects the entire zone. Every part, gland, or organ of the body represented in a particular zone can be stimulated by working on any reflex in that same zone.

In addition to the longitudinal zones of CZT, reflexology also uses the transverse zones (horizontal zones) on the body and feet or hands. The purpose is to help fix the image of the body by mapping it onto the hands or feet in proper perspective and location. Four transverse zone lines are commonly used: transverse pelvic line, transverse waistline, transverse diaphragm line, and transverse neck line. These transverse zone lines create five areas: pelvic area, lower abdominal area, upper abdominal area, thoracic area, and head area.

Internal organs layer on top, over, behind, between, and against each other in every possible configuration. The reflexes on the hands and feet that correspond to the parts, organs, and glands, overlap as well.

A basic premise of CZT is that the right foot or hand represents the right side of the body, and the left foot or hand, the left side. However, in the nervous system, the right half of the brain controls the left side of the body, and vice versa. In any disorders that affect the brain or the central nervous system, a reflexologist will emphasize the reflexes or areas of the disorder on the opposite hand or foot. For example, the brain reflexes are worked on the left foot or hand for strokes that caused paralysis on the right side of the body.

Although it is commonly assumed that the hands and feet are the only areas to which reflexology can be applied, there are reflexes throughout the ten zones of the body that present seemingly unlikely relations within each zone. For example, there is a zonal relationship between the eyes and the kidneys, because both lie in the same zone. Working the kidney reflexes can affect the eyes.

If there is an injury on the foot, the area should be avoided and should not be worked, and alternate parts of the body in the same zone may be worked instead. For example, the arm is a reflection of the leg, the hand of the foot, the wrist of the ankle, and so forth. If any part of the arm is injured, the corresponding part of the leg can be worked, and vice versa. Common problems such as varicose veins and phlebitis in the legs can be helped by working the same general areas on the arms.

This approach can be used to find referral areas by identifying the zone(s) in which an injury has occurred and tracing it to the referral area. Tenderness in the referral area will usually help to locate it.

Referral areas can give insights into a problem by indicating areas in the same zone(s) that may be at the root of the problem. For example, a shoulder problem may be related to a hip problem, since the shoulder lies in the same zone as the hip. These relations may be understood biomechanically as well as energetically.

A reflexology session usually begins on the right foot or hand and finishes on the left foot or hand. In addition, the reflexes on both feet and hands are worked from the base of the foot or hand up to the top, with the toes or fingers worked last.

Feedback control

For self-regulation of the body, a highly complex and integrated communication control system or network operates as a "feedback control loop." Different networks in the body control diverse functions, such as blood carbon dioxide levels, temperature, and heart and respiratory rates. Homeostatic control mechanisms are categorized as *negative or positive feedback loops*. Many of the important and numerous homeostatic control mechanisms are negative feedback loops.

Negative feedback loops are stabilizing mechanisms. For example, they maintain homeostasis of blood carbon dioxide concentration. As blood carbon dioxide increases, the respiration rate increases to permit increased amounts of carbon dioxide to exit the body through expired air. Without this homeostatic mechanism, body carbon dioxide levels would rapidly rise to toxic levels, and death would result.

The blood circulation loop is from the left side of the body to the right side—fresh oxygenated blood enters the aorta from the left ventricle of the heart and travels to the body, and venous blood with carbon dioxide enters the vena cava on the right side of the heart. By beginning a reflexology session on the right foot or hand, the reflexologist is helping to boost the loop by pushing venous or deoxygenated blood into the heart and lungs so that fresh oxygenated blood will be available to the body cells. The same rationale applies to the direction in which the reflexologist works on the foot or hand—from the bottom upward, to bolster the homeostatic loop.

Reflexology demonstrates four main benefits:

1. It promotes relaxation by the removal of stress.

2. It enhances circulation.

3. It assists the body to normalize metabolism naturally.

4. It complements other healing modalities.

When the reflexes are stimulated, the body's natural energy works along the nervous system to clear any blockages in the corresponding zones.

A reflexology session seems to break up deposits (felt as a sandy or gritty area under the skin) which may interfere with the flow of the body's electrical energy in the nervous system.

In clinical studies, reflexology has been found to be effective in reducing pain in women with severe premenstrual symptoms and in patients with migraine and tension headaches. It has also demonstrated benefit in alleviating motor, sensory, and urinary symptoms in patients with multiple sclerosis. Recent reviews on the efficacy of reflexology in cancer patients found positive improvements in anxiety and pain. The adverse effects of reflexology are minor and may include fatigue (increase in parasympathetic activity), headache, nausea, increased perspiration, and diarrhea.

Reflexology impacts the autonomic nervous system more directly than many other therapies, balancing the parasympathetic nervous system and the sympathetic nervous system, the two subdivisions of the autonomic nervous system that exert opposite effects on the end organs, to maintain or restore homeostasis—and so it can be seen that the well-known concept of homeostasis in Western scientific medicine and physiology has its equivalent in the ancient concept of *balance* as the goal of Chinese medical therapies.

For practitioners, certification is provided by certain educational institutions. There are many schools of reflexology that can provide adequate training, ranging from 100 to 1000 hours of instruction. The interested individual should look for a school that is established and, if possible, recognized by a local governing body. In the United States and Canada, there are regulations for practicing reflexology, and some individual states and provinces (though not all) have their own sets of educational or licensing requirements.

Qi gong and t'ai chi (qi cultivation)

Vital energy or qi may also be influenced by other means without specific reference to acupuncture points, channels, or meridians, as in the practice of qi gong.

Qi gong, or *qi* cultivation, encompasses a broad range of practices and activities including the meditative systems of *Daoist* and *Buddhist* practitioners, the health-giving exercises developed by *ancient physicians*, and the *martial arts* traditions of China. The common feature of these practices is the intention of *enhancing qi*—by allowing the individual to increase its quantity, smooth its flow, and place it under a greater degree of conscious control, thereby strengthening the *body, energy, mind,* and *spirit.*

While Daoist and Buddhist *qi gong* focus on *spiritual* realization, *medical qi* cultivation addresses three areas. The first is *self-cultivation,* or the development of the practitioner's own health and stamina. The second involves the cultivation of the practitioner's ability to safely *transmit qi* to the patient, either by means of needles or directly through the hands. The third is *teaching patients* to perform specific *qi gong* practices to address particular health issues or generally strengthen their *qi.*

How qi gong works

"Flowing water will never turn stale, the hinge of the door will never be eaten by worms," explains *Lu's Spring and Autumn Annals.* "They never rest in their activity: that's why."

Qi cultivation is a very ancient part of traditional Chinese medicine. The texts recovered at Ma Huang Dui include illustrated guides to therapeutic properties and physical practices of a form of *qi gong* known as conduction (*Dao yin*). In the second century, Hua Tou created a series of exercises based on the movements of the tiger, deer, bear, monkey, and bird, which were practiced to ward off disease.

Qi gong has many forms of practice, which can be performed standing, sitting, or lying down, but always involves *relaxation of the body, regulation of the breath,* and *calming of the mind.*

One form of *qi gong* involves visualizing internal and external pathways of the channels and imagining *qi* moving along them in concert with the breath. As the practice develops, the practitioner begins to experience the sensation of *qi* traveling along the channel pathways. The mind guides *qi* to a specific area of the body, then the *qi* guides blood to that same area, improving circulation. This exercise is designed to train *qi* and blood to move freely along the channel pathways, leading to good health.

Another exercise, often recommended for people with bronchitis, emphysema, or bronchial asthma, involves the use of breathing, visualization, and simple physical exercises to benefit the *qi* of the lungs. Assuming a relaxed posture, the practitioner begins by breathing naturally and allowing the mind to become calm. The upper and lower teeth are then gently clicked together 36 times. As saliva is produced, it is retained in the mouth, swirled with the tongue, then swallowed in three parts while imagining that it is flowing into the middle of the chest and then to an area about three finger-widths below the navel (the *dan tian* or "cinnabar field"). At this point, the practitioner imagines sitting in front of a reservoir of white *qi*, which enters the mouth on the inhalation, and is transmitted through the body on the exhalation, first to the lungs, then to the *dan tian*, and finally out to the skin and body hair. This process of visualization is repeated 18 times.

These exercises may sound odd to Westerners, but they have been used for many centuries to enhance breathing, circulation, and other vital bodily functions, as well as to address the individual's mental and spiritual state. The cultivation of *qi* is an integral part of traditional Chinese medicine, both within China and throughout the world.

In these ways, *qi gong* is one of the most ancient yet modern, profound yet simple applications of the celestial (spiritual) healing and vital energy of Chinese medicine.

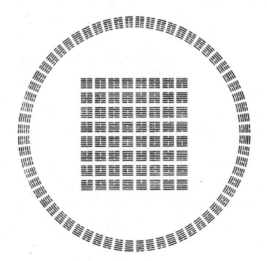

Figure 7.1 The 64 Hexagrams of I Ching

PART II

❧

East Asia

Chapter 8

Korean and Japanese Medicine

Both Korean and Japanese medicine utilize the concept of *gi*, or *ki*, based on early translations of Chinese medical texts and the introduction of medical practitioners to their courts.

Adoption of Chinese medical theory and *materia medica* took place sooner on the *Korean Peninsula*, due largely to its geographical location adjacent to the Chinese empire. During the Song Dynasty (970–1279), medical texts such as the *Suwen* were imported to the Koryo Court of Korea (see Chapter 2). Early forms of Korean medicine extensively utilized Chinese medical theories of yin (陰) and yang (陽), meridians, acupuncture, and *qi*. Later forms of Korean medicine evolved with (1) herbal medicine *indigenous* to the area, and (2) charismatic *Buddhist* monks who focused on healing. Eventually a *hybrid* system of knowledge utilizing Chinese medical concepts of vital energy, together with local medicinal plants, became the foundation of traditional *Korean* medicine.

As with Chinese medicine, famous doctors known for their techniques and writings were key figures in promulgating the spread of medical beliefs and practice through texts.

Political relations between China and Korea were close during the period of the development of medicine in China when Chinese medicine arrived in Korea during the Qin Dynasty (221–207 BCE). However, the textual basis of Korean medicine, in the literary tradition of Chinese medicine, appears to have been established in the Han and Tang dynasties during a period of political domination by the Chinese. Continuing close relations between China and Korea during the Korean Kingdom of Silla (400–700 CE) facilitated this exchange of ideas.

Formal medical instruction by government-appointed physicians began in 693 CE. Texts such as the *Systematic Classic of Acupuncture* were important to the development of the tradition. With the formation of the Korean Liao Dynasty (907–1168), Korea established its independence from Chinese rule, but cultural and medical exchange continued. During the Korean Li Dynasty (1392–1910) many Chinese texts, including the *Illustrated Classic of Acupuncture Points as Found on the Bronze Model*, reached Korea.

Widely used techniques of acupuncture point selection based on *Five Phase Theory* emerged from Korea, including those of the *Buddhist* priest Sa-am (1544–1610).

Korean innovations

At least two relatively recent innovations based on Chinese medicine were developed in Korea and have become well known in other parts of the world. *Korean constitutional diagnosis* was a system of herbal therapeutics developed initially by Jhema Lee (1836–1900). It was elaborated subsequently by Dowon Kuan who, in 1965, expanded the system to an eightfold classification and applied it to acupuncture (Hirsch 1985)—compare Ayurvedic constitutional types, or *Doshas* (see Micozzi 2011).

Another influential contemporary system is that of *Koryo Sooji Chim*, the system of Korean hand and finger acupuncture developed by Yoo Tae Woo in 1971. It maps the channel pathways and acupuncture points of the entire body onto the hands, where they are stimulated using very short, fine needles and magnets. This system has gained a significant level of international exposure.

Japan

While the history of cultural exchange between China and Japan dates back to at least 57 CE, Chinese medicine was introduced to Japan only during the fifth and sixth centuries, through a range of travelers between the two countries, including court emissaries, physicians and *Buddhist* monks. Chinese Song Dynasty medical texts were a key part of this transmission of knowledge. As with Korean medicine, Japanese integration of Chinese medicine incorporated the basic medical concepts of vital energy, *ki*, and *yin–yang* balance. Premodern medical texts such as the *Ishimpo* (*Methods at the Heart of Medicine*) and Menase Dosan's 15-volume, sixteenth-century medical text, utilize these concepts in their discussion of diseases and their treatment.

Japanese medicine was influenced not only by Chinese medical theory but also by *Buddhist* and *Zen* practitioners, and from the late eighteenth century onwards by Western medical knowledge introduced by the Dutch and Germans. Traditional Japanese medicine also evolved to develop specialized knowledge of acupressure (*shiatsu*), distinct techniques in acupuncture, bone manipulation, and setting techniques (see Chapter 10).

Chinese physicians in ancient Japan

Kon Mu was the first physician using Chinese methods to come to Japan. He was sent in 414 CE by the King of Silla, in Southeast Korea, to treat the Emperor Inkyo Tenno. This interaction continued in 552 with a Korean delegation which brought a selection of Chinese medical texts to Japan. In 562 Zhi Cong came from southern China with more than 100 books on the practice of Chinese medicine, including the *Systematic Classic of Acupuncture*. By the early eighth century the influence of Chinese medicine was well established. In 702, provision was made for a ministry of health composed of specialists, physicians, students, and researchers. In 754 a Buddhist priest, Chien Chen, brought many medical texts from China to Japan.

Japanese revisions

Chinese influences on Japanese medicine were originally derived primarily from the *Classic of Difficult Issues* and *Systematic Classic of Acupuncture*. A revisionist movement in the late seventeenth century established the *Treatise on Cold Damage* (*Shokanron*), perhaps better reflecting the native climate of Japan, as the core text of herbal medicine, or *kampo* (Chinese method), in Japan.

Several factors have influenced the development of Chinese medicine in Japan, giving it a somewhat unique appearance. The scarcity of natural resources and ingredients in the islands of Japan limited the preparation of Chinese herbal formulas and led to an emphasis on herbal prescriptions *in lower doses* than are typical in China. An emphasis on *palpatory diagnosis* involving channel pathways and the abdomen also became well established. The use of somewhat finer-gauge needles and shallow insertion became typical of Japanese acupuncture.

Blind acupuncture, shiatsu and massage

It became customary in the earlier part of the Japanese Edo period (1603–1868) for massage to be done by blind practitioners. Practice by blind masseurs, thought to be more skilled due to their heightened sense of touch and other non-visual senses, had originated in China. Blindness was also useful in the practice, since it was considered taboo to look upon a woman's naked body. (To avoid touching women, female patients would indicate the site of their problems on an anatomical doll instead of on their own bodies, and physicians would attach fine silk threads to women's wrists so that they could detect a pulse from behind a curtain, or even in another room.)

In Japan, embarrassment was further avoided by performing massage through loose-fitting clothing. In the mid-seventeenth century, Waichi Sugiyama, a blind man, began to train the blind in acupuncture, using very fine needles and guide tubes. In this way both massage and acupuncture became associated with blind practitioners. Combining the two approaches, Japanese practice used application of manual pressure on acupuncture points (see Chapter 7). Chinese *anma* (from the Chinese word for massage) was replaced by a formalized system of *shiatsu*—*shi* meaning finger, and *atsu*, pressure, in Japanese.

These occupations undertaken by the blind contributed to a lower social ranking of acupuncture practitioners, and to the segmentation and specialization of medical practice in Japan.

Kampo medicine

During the development of medicine in Japan, *kampo*, or *kanpo*, physicians became primarily practitioners of herbal medicine. Today the integrated form of Chinese medicine in Japan is referred to as *kampo* (漢方). Like its traditional Chinese medicine (TCM) counterpart, *kampo* has integrated evidence-based research and Western biomedical concepts. For example, *ki* in contemporary *kampo* is described, very much in twentieth-century terms, as a vital energy that allows the mind and body to function appropriately, and which may correspond to activities of the central nervous system and autonomic nervous system. The functioning of *ki* can be disturbed by psychosocial stressors.

Japanese medical specialization

This trend toward specialization has continued to the present day, with the division of acupuncture, moxibustion, and massage into separately licensed practices (although many individuals hold all three licenses), and the actual practice of herbal medicine being retained in the hands of medical doctors as a form of internal medicine. Accordingly, Chinese herbal prescriptions are recognized as appropriate therapy for certain medical conditions, according to regulations governing health care in Japan.

Japanese medical renaissance

Japan has seen both focused specialization in, and innovative exploration and expansion of, traditional acupuncture. The *Classic of Difficult Issues* has often been the focus for movements to revive the practices of traditional acupuncture. Its influence has contributed heavily to the comparatively recent development of groups of acupuncturists advocating *meridian therapy* (*keiraku chiryo*) based on the application of vital energy concepts in the *Classic of Difficult Issues* and their subsequent interpretation by later Chinese authors. A distinctive feature of meridian therapy is the application of *Five Phase Theory* to the transport points, a practice that also influenced the ultimate perception and adoption of Five Phase Theory in the popular form of Chinese medicine utilized by European practitioners.

The pioneering work of Yoshio Manaka also contributed dramatically to the practice of acupuncture. Manaka, a physician who experimented with acupuncture principles during a *period when medical supplies were absent in World War II* (see also Chapters 15 and 16), became convinced of the efficacy and physiological relevance of traditional theories and continued to experiment and develop them throughout his life.

The range of practices and interests of Japanese acupuncture practitioners is quite broad. While some are particular partisans of specific schools of thought, including some based on contemporary Chinese medical perspectives, many Japanese practitioners have adopted a comparatively eclectic approach.

Chapter 9

✿

Macrobiotics

Originating in early twentieth-century Japan, macrobiotics is now a widely used alternative nutritional approach in Europe and the United States. A macrobiotic diet is primarily vegetarian, high in complex carbohydrates, and low in fat. Macrobiotics also offers a *spiritual* philosophy embraced to varying degrees by many thousands of practitioners around the world. Michio Kushi is an influential macrobiotic teacher who has made significant claims for the success of macrobiotics in treating cancer and other chronic diseases.

In its current manifestation, macrobiotics originated in Japan in the late nineteenth and early twentieth centuries with an educator named Yukikazu Sakurazawa and a physician named Sagen Ishisuka. They reportedly cured themselves of serious illnesses by changing from a modern, refined diet to a traditional Japanese simple diet of brown rice, miso soup, sea vegetables, and other traditional Japanese foods. After restoring their health, they went on to integrate traditional *Oriental medicine and philosophy* with *Vedanta* (a Hindu spiritual tradition), original Judeo-Christian teachings, and holistic perspectives in modern science and medicine. Some critics have asserted that Sakurazawa and Ishisuka never intended this theological base, and that later proponents of macrobiotics, particularly

Michio Kushi, were responsible for the spiritual element. When Sakurazawa came to Paris in the 1920s he adopted the pseudonym George Ohsawa, and called his teachings "macrobiotics." The word "macrobiotics" is derived from the Greek *macro*, meaning "great" or "large," and *bios*, "life."

Before leaving Japan, Kushi studied briefly with George Ohsawa. It was Ohsawa's belief that food was the key to health. By returning to a traditional diet of whole, natural foods, he believed that humanity could regain its physical and mental balance. While living in New York, Kushi experienced positive changes in his own health and consciousness after changing his own diet. Over the next ten years, with the support of his wife Aveline, he began to study traditional and modern approaches to diet and health and to teach macrobiotics.

In the 1960s, Kushi moved to Boston and founded Erewhon (one of the early natural foods distributors) to make available the foods necessary for a macrobiotic lifestyle. In 1971, his followers founded *East–West Journal*, and the following year the East–West Foundation was started to support macrobiotic education and research. In 1978, Michio and Aveline Kushi founded the Kushi Institute, with affiliated organizations throughout Europe. Aveline died in 2001 of cancer at a relatively young age.

In the 1970s Kushi decided to present macrobiotics with a major emphasis on its role in the prevention and alleviation of cancer. His son, Lawrence Kushi, PhD, a respected nutrition researcher, has commented that macrobiotics was generally seen in its role as a *philosophy* of life. Later it became most widely known as a *cancer diet*. Michio Kushi moved in that direction. Some would ask whether that was the right decision, or whether cancer was necessarily the right disease to promote it, since a macrobiotic diet has not been scientifically demonstrated to be effective with cancer.

Macrobiotics and similar vegetarian diets are arguably preventive for those cancers most closely associated with a high-fat Western diet, although this relationship is not clear. These diets may some day prove to be effective for patients with some types of cancer, in the inhibition or reversal of tumor progression as well as in the extension of remission and overall survival after surgical or medical treatment. However, at the time of writing, well-designed scientific research has yet to determine whether, and in what ways, macrobiotics is helpful with cancer.

Kushi makes a number of observations from history and contemporary science to support his view that (1) a grain-based diet can inhibit cancer and permit the patient to survive longer; (2) artificial infant feeding is associated with increased incidence of breast cancer among mothers; (3) caloric restriction results in reduced incidence of cancer in animals; and (4) a vegetarian diet prevents breast cancer. The author of this book has also reviewed and presented compelling evidence (Micozzi 1986) that supports points (2) and (3), with some support for point (4) but no support for point (1) above. Unfortunately, from the standpoint of macrobiotics, point (1) is a cornerstone of the whole approach.

Dietary recommendations

Kushi's dietary recommendations may provide a healthy and nutritionally balanced diet, but are based on a complex macrobiotic dietary theory that has no foundation in scientific medicine. The specific foods included and excluded by macrobiotics for cancer differ from those recommended by other dietary systems based on traditional Asian medicine. Macrobiotic dietary theory is unproven from a mainstream medical perspective, and in many respects contradicts other traditional dietary regimens, such as naturopathic or Ayurvedic dietary programs. Ayurvedic medicine from India, for example, gives dietary recommendations for cancer that are quite different from, and often contradict, macrobiotic recommendations. Likewise, the evidence from Western medicine is also largely contradictory (Micozzi 2007). Systems of traditional medicine differ in detail, but generally recommend fresh, whole foods. Kushi's recommendation of seaweed (sea vegetables) is supported by suggestive scientific evidence.

Cancer cure?

Kushi does not call his approach a cancer cure. While he gives examples of patients who reportedly recovered from metastatic or otherwise life-threatening cancers using macrobiotics, the cases often include explicit evidence that misdiagnosis might have been involved, or that the case was not entirely hopeless from a mainstream perspective. By avoiding the representation of macrobiotics as a cancer cure, Kushi has avoided serious conflict with mainstream medicine.

Other groups of practitioners who have avoided serious conflict with mainstream medicine are practitioners of traditional *Chinese* medicine. They have often been more cautious than Kushi, and make no special claims about cancer. Many practitioners even refuse to treat cancer; and those who do emphasize the purely adjunctive nature of their treatment. As a result, tens of thousands of American cancer patients avail themselves of the supportive treatment of traditional Chinese medicine. Strategic placement of treatments outside the medical mainstream is one of the skills of Asian culture, accustomed to taking the long view and to achieving goals by indirect means when direct confrontation would be counterproductive.

Case histories, physician reports, and scientific studies that relate to the use of macrobiotics in cancer are sketchy. They do suggest that macrobiotics may have, at least, some positive impact for some people with cancer. One of the most credible independent advocates of a macrobiotic approach to cancer was Anthony Sattilaro, MD (1982), whose book *Recalled by Life* describes his recovery from metastatic prostatic cancer. He underwent conventional therapy, but his physician told him that he had at best only a few years to live. He then turned to macrobiotics, experienced a spiritual awakening, and subsequently recovered. The story of his recovery did for macrobiotics something akin to what the story of *New York Times* columnist James Reston's experience in China did for acupuncture (see pages 197–199).

Macrobiotics brought an alternative therapy to public attention through a single personal account. Sattilaro was chief medical executive of Methodist Hospital in Philadelphia, having previously served as chairman of the anesthesiology department. After his initial recovery using macrobiotics, Sattilaro distanced himself from the macrobiotic movement, especially from its more spiritual components and its belief system. But his belief in the importance of his own spiritual awakening and the whole-food vegetarian diet persisted. Sattilaro died of a recurrence of his cancer in 1989.

Takeshi Hirayama of the National Cancer Research Institute in Japan reported in 1982 that daily intake of soybean (*miso*) soup correlated with dramatically reduced gastric cancer rates in a large-scale prospective study of over 260,000 Japanese men and women. The standardized mortality rates for men who drank miso soup daily was 172 per 100,000 compared to a rate of 256 for men who never drank miso soup, with intermediate values for men who drank miso soup occasionally or rarely. The rates for women were 78 for daily miso soup drinkers and 114 for women who never drank miso soup. Hirayama noted that the results could be due to the effects of beneficial compounds such as protease inhibitors or other nutritional factors in the soybean paste, or of other beneficial foods that frequently accompany soybean soup, such as green and yellow vegetables.

Two studies on *seaweeds* used in macrobiotics are of interest. Teas and colleagues (1984) looked at the possibility that brown seaweed (kelp), which is widely consumed by Japanese women, could be prophylactic for carcinogen-induced mammary tumors in rats. Experimental rats fed kelp took almost twice as long to develop tumors as the control rats, and had a 13 percent reduction in the number of cancers that developed. A second seaweed study, by Tanka and colleagues, looked at the role of polysaccharides from brown seaweed (kelp) in inhibiting the intestinal absorption of radioactive strontium.

The macrobiotic program is clearly not a definitive cure for cancer. If it were, the researchers who gathered cases for analysis would have found more examples.

On the other hand, there are a considerable number of well-documented, unexpected recoveries, including recoveries from metastatic cancers. The available data suggest that the kind of person who chooses the rigors of the macrobiotic program may be likely, for psychological reasons, to have a more optimistic outlook regarding quality of life and survival, apart from possible effects of the diet, and that the effect of this might be in the range of doubling the length of survival, which is the same as the rate reported for a number of psychological interventions.

Many believe that it is not the macrobiotic diet per se that has an anti-cancer effect, but probably any healthy diet that does not contain substantial amounts of dairy food.

It is surprising that the macrobiotic community has produced so little in the way of definitive research on the effects of macrobiotics on cancer. The available evidence suggests that macrobiotics may be of moderate help in certain people with some types of cancer. However, when we consider the biological adaptation of the human organism, it would be somewhat surprising to find a diet so heavily based upon grains (relative latecomers in human dietary history) to be particularly healthy. The effect of the "hard fibers" in grains might also be found to promote cellular division in the gastrointestinal tract and to promote gastrointestinal cancers, for example. On the whole, a physician might be reluctant to endorse macrobiotics in the prevention or management of cancer, based upon current evidence and understanding of nutrition and cancer.

Chapter 10

Reiki and Shiatsu

Reiki

Reiki, in the same way as macrobiotics, had its origin in Japan in the 1920s and was exported to the West later in the twentieth century and adapted for Western use. However, like ancient Chinese medicine, it is said to date back to earlier times. Reiki is also ascribed semi-mythical origins which are projected back onto historically ancient practices. Unlike Chinese medicine, on the other hand, contemporary Reiki is very much a product of the twentieth century whose popularity has been bolstered by the New Age.

"Reiki" is translated from Japanese as "universal life energy." As a method of hands-on healing, it is handed down orally from master to student. Many different schools, or *streams*, as they are called in the present-day Japanese view, developed from the original teachings of Mikao Usui in the early 1920s.

Shinto roots

The roots of Usui's System of Natural Healing (as it is called) have been superimposed on those of Shintoism, an early religion of Japanese peoples prior to acculturation to China. Shintoism itself had no formal organization until it was used as a political tool to enhance the lineage of the Meiji Emperors and Meiji Restoration. As practiced in its earliest form (200 BCE), it included belief in spirit beings and the energy of every living thing, as well as in entities that the Western mind finds difficult to believe are animate, such as stones and waterfalls.

Reiki can be understood in its fullest capacity when linked with the Shinto worldview, which recognizes elemental spiritual forces and energy. However, the system is also said to rely on Buddhist tradition introduced from China, in some of its practices, in regarding the world and its elements as transient. Further, there are Christian charismatic elements which might be seen as apt for the cultural era of 1920s Japan as it emerged into the twentieth century (prior to becoming isolated in the militarism of the 1930s and World War II).

According to the "creation myth" of modern Reiki, Dr. Mikao Usui was searching for concrete ways in which Jesus and the Buddha were able to heal with the "laying on of hands." Oral histories agree that the point of origin for this system occurred when Dr. Usui undertook a lengthy meditation and fast on Mount Kuiyama outside Kyoto, Japan, and received information, guidance, and initiation into this healing modality.

Dr. Usui began teaching his method in 1920, and one year later he opened a Reiki practice in Harajuko, Tokyo, close to the Meiji Jinju. Dr. Usui developed and taught five spiritual precepts as guidelines for everyday living and foci for personal meditation. Followers disagree about the basis of these precepts. Some believe they are based on the Meiji Emperor's "five rules of life." Others believe these writings were developed as positive reflections of the five hindrances to spiritual enlightenment presented by the Buddha.

Several Reiki lineages have grown out of the original teachings of Dr. Usui. A Hawaiian-born, Japanese–American woman, Hawayo Takata, began teaching Reiki to the West in the 1970s. Her story is widely known because it has been chronicled in many books and retold throughout the world.

Many schools have developed which have varying requirements in training, but all hold as true that the transfer of energy, Reiki, from one human being to another living being is real. There is a growing number of anecdotal accounts regarding the rebalancing of mind, body, and spirit and the release of disease or pain as a result of Reiki treatment.

Research is beginning to be done on this system as a valid therapy, and the Usui system of Reiki is being taught to nurses in hospitals and in nursing schools. Doctors, dentists, psychologists, and other health care providers are learning this technique to add a "hands-on" dimension of calming, healing touch to their practices.

Now there are manuals and written texts, cassettes and videos, discussing a wide array of personal interpretations of this system. But techniques of application are diverse, as they depend on the oral teachings of each master as he or she initiated and instructed students. Not until the Usui system itself faced competition from other emerging Reiki schools and styles was there any attempt by a professional organization to establish a systematic approach. The Reiki Alliance was originally formed to support the teachings of Hawayo Takata through her granddaughter Phyllis Furumoto. In 1993 it began to define qualifications and ethical standards for Reiki practice. Several organizations have subsequently developed their own criteria to promote wider acceptance.

Healing what needs to be healed

Most Reiki practitioners are not concerned with a client's medical diagnosis unless they are coordinating with a doctor or other medical provider. Reiki supports healing only of what needs to be healed, rather than what the practitioner intends to be healed. For this reason, Reiki practitioners generally do not promise any specific symptom improvement or "cure."

Sometimes only one session is needed, and sometimes multiple sessions are needed for clients to begin to realize they are experiencing shifts in their perspective on life, and on the nature of their disease, as well as in their attitudes and in the nature of the symptoms that brought them into the treatment in the first place.

Part of Reiki's effectiveness can be attributed to the body's response to gentle, appropriate contact between practitioner and client. The practitioner gains permission to touch the client, then places his or her hands in a prescribed pattern on the client's body. The client is clothed and may be standing, sitting, or reclining on a bed, massage table, or the floor.

Many compare the feeling of receiving Reiki to the sensation felt when praying, meditating, singing, walking in the woods, or in any other way actively seeking the presence of God. Many Reiki practitioners believe these sensations are the physical responses to making a connection with a power greater than themselves. Students are assisted in becoming aware (again) of the Universal Energy, that is, "a life force that abounds in everything," and that human beings benefit when they remain open to it.

The body automatically directs healing energy to wounds, strain, tension, and other ailments. It is believed a person receiving Reiki draws this energy through the hands of the practitioner, who is open to its universal availability. The hands are simply placed over an area of pain, infection or tension, and the mind is opened and energy is allowed to flow. There is no manipulation of muscles or of the "electromagnetic field" of a client. The only method is to apply touch to a client's body in the prescribed hand positions and/or to be guided by an intuitive force. Some schools of Reiki do not allow the practitioner's hands to touch the client's body. The origin of this practice is not clear; traditional practitioners use this "hands-off" technique only when treating open or fresh wounds caused by accident or surgery. Some schools of Reiki teach that the practitioner's hands should remain in place for a period of three to five minutes. The traditional practitioner leaves the hands in position until the flow of energy is no longer felt.

For any condition, the basic routine is to offer a full body treatment session and then return to the site of the original pain, stress, or tension. However, case reports indicate that after applying the full body treatment, a practitioner has no need to return to the original area of complaint because the problem has already been resolved.

When a practitioner places hands on a client, both the practitioner and the client observe sensory changes around or under the hands of the practitioner. These changes include the sensations of warmth, tingling, cold, extra fullness, and electrical charge. These sensations can change from one day to the next, from one client to the next, and can be experienced differently by the practitioner and the client. These sensory changes indicate that something is passing between the practitioner and the client. When the sensation dissipates after a time of holding the hands in one position, it signals to the practitioner to change hand positions; in other words, to move on. There is no conscious effort needed on the part of a practitioner to "turn Reiki on." When the body is in pain, has sustained a wound, or is beset by an unbalanced glandular, metabolic, or enzymatic process, it gives out an electromagnetic, neural, atomic, or vibrational alarm to stimulate a healing response from the rest of the body. How else does the body's immune system send its cells to repel intruding bacteria, or platelets to a wound to help stop bleeding? If we could record this signal with sensitive diagnostic equipment, we would understand the call of the body for internal or external energy. The fact that the sensation of Reiki energy flow dissipates after a time tells us that the particular need has been satisfied for the time being. The time-frame for this shift may be as little as a few seconds or as long as 45 minutes, or until the practitioner tires of holding the position.

The phenomenon of energy exchange can also explain the intuitive experience of many practitioners who find their hands drawn to a particular part of the client's body. The practitioner has no conscious knowledge of where the client is holding tension. It has been explained that the energy itself (meaning Reiki) feels the call of the body and is drawn to the need.

Intentionality in healing

In the recent proliferation of anecdotes in books and on the Internet, no harmful effects of Reiki have been reported. One of the issues frequently discussed is the role of the *intent* of the practitioner. It is most often agreed that the only necessary intent is to be available to channel the energy, rather than to "heal" a certain symptom or condition. Clients are often healed in unexpected ways. For this reason, traditional Reiki practitioners make no promises regarding the efficacy of treatment. Many practitioners, seeking to avoid any promise of therapeutic value, refer to the hour-long applications of energy simply as "sessions" or "therapy appointments."

The many anecdotal testimonies show Reiki to support the natural healing process of the body to such an extent that it can stimulate what is called a *healing crisis* (a term originally coined in homeopathy)—for example bringing a boil to a head, thus allowing the wound to be cleaned; or a sudden rise in temperature in someone with an infection, followed by a gradual return to normal. Some practitioners have reported that cuts, surgical wounds, and broken bones healed faster than expected after applying Reiki. There is also anecdotal evidence of Reiki resulting in reduction of the side effects of chemotherapy and radiation treatment.

Reiki is often described as working on the root cause of a disease or imbalance. If a mental, emotional, or spiritual disturbance is a major factor in a physical impairment, the client often recognizes the disturbance during a Reiki session. How to deal with a painful relationship or a financial problem can be revealed during a session. As stated earlier, healing can come in many forms.

When practitioners or others who have been attuned to Reiki regularly apply this energy to themselves, they experience a dramatic reduction in daily stress levels. When energy application is coupled with focused attention, through "processing work," or meditation on the five precepts, personal understanding and an increase in compassion and openness to life can also occur.

People who have attended classes describe personal experiences that defy logical explanation. These experiences are designated as mystical, synchronistic, or even *cosmic*. Because they are often very personal, these experiences are not referred to in medically oriented classes, so as not to put off clinicians who require concrete explanations.

Treatment styles

European treatment styles differ from those taught in *American* schools. Some teach more hand positions, and often offer the application of Reiki to clients who are covered with only a sheet or blanket. Other styles of Reiki application are not described in relation to body organs. Traditional Japanese anatomy, like Chinese, is based on energetic relationships and not upon anatomical dissection or the physical locations of the organs as known to Western medicine. For example, one school of Reiki designates a series of hand positions in relation to *chakras*, energy centers, in a line from the pubic bone to the top of the head. This chakra system is derived from Vedic philosophy and was not in the original teachings of the Usui system.

Three degrees of Reiki

Traditionally there have been three levels or degrees in the Usui system.

First degree Reiki

First degree (Reiki I) is often referred to as "beginning Reiki." This label may lead a person to believe that he or she has to take the next levels in order to have a complete understanding of Reiki, or to be able to fully use the Usui system of natural healing. In the traditional system, Reiki I is sufficient to become a Reiki practitioner or to offer Reiki to oneself and family members for health maintenance and stress prevention.

This class is taught in three four-hour sessions and includes four initiations or "attunements," which are the methods of connecting an individual with the source of energy. Once connected to that source, a student is connected for life. During this class, students are taught the history of Reiki, observe the hand positions, and are invited to give and experience a full body application. Discussion of the five precepts is encouraged. Students are also encouraged to experience self-treatment and to investigate the application of Reiki in emergency situations, in hospices or hospitals, and to clients with acute or chronic conditions. Many case studies are reviewed and the dynamic potential of having access to this energy is outlined. Often students experience changes in their health, their relationships, or other human conditions during this training. The only prerequisites for learning are openness, a desire to learn, and a commitment to use Reiki regularly.

Second degree Reiki

Second degree (Reiki II) is referred to in some schools as Advanced Training. It involves instruction in additional applications of Reiki through the use of symbols or energy patterns. These additional applications include being able to offer Reiki to a person who is not in the room. This person can be nextdoor or on the other side of the globe. The technique is called "sending Reiki" or "distant Reiki" and is akin to distant healing. Another application is that of mental rebalancing, which involves a specific hand position and techniques to help relieve addictions and habits and also to improve mental clarity. A third application is the ability to focus Reiki into a laser-like beam or to intensify its concentration. This class is taught over two days, or a minimum of two sessions. Often a Reiki master asks a student to return in a month to share experiences regarding practice at this level of application.

Third degree Reiki

Third degree (Reiki III), or Master Training, may last as long as a year. Some schools have divided this training into two additional levels, Third Degree and Master Teacher Training, while others have consolidated this training into a one-day experience. Many agree that this level of training can be taxing on the person who wishes to pursue this degree of commitment. According to the Reiki Alliance, a student of Reiki should have been actively working with Reiki for three to ten years before moving into this level of training.

A person who completes this training has the knowledge and technique with which to educate and open others to Reiki. How to initiate others into all three degrees is only one part of this mastery. Several organizations have developed teaching protocols for all levels of training. Each master may add his or her own requirements.

All three levels are taught by a master who has fulfilled all training requirements. They are known as *Reiki masters*, not because they have mastered the energy, but because they have made a commitment to "stand in the light of Reiki" and allow their lives to "exemplify the qualities described in the five precepts." This commitment is made on many levels, including the financial, political, emotional, and spiritual.

Shiatsu

The literal meaning of the Japanese word *shiatsu* is "finger pressure" or "thumb pressure." The practice of massage dates back 3000 years in China. *Shiatsu* is seen to have antecedents in Chinese medicine—for example, in the 2000-year-old *Yellow Emperor's Classic of Internal Medicine*, and over the centuries Chinese medicine and massage therapy, as well as twentieth-century advancements, have combined to yield "modern" *shiatsu* (Palanjian 2002).

As a healing art or treatment it grew from earlier forms of *anma* in Japan and *tui na* in China (see Chapter 7). *An* denotes "pressure" and *ma* means "rubbing." This method, well known in China, found its way to Japan and became recognized as a safe and easy way to treat the human body. In Japan, a tradition developed for *shiatsu* to be used and taught by blind practitioners who relied on their hands to diagnose a patient's condition (see Chapter 8).

Anma was recognized as a medical modality in Japan during the Nara period (710–784), but subsequently lost its popularity before gaining more widespread use in the Edo era (1603–1868), during which doctors were required to study Anma. During the Edo period, most practitioners were blind and provided treatments in their patients' homes. *Anma*'s understanding and assessment of human structure and meridian lines were, and are, believed to be important distinctions that separate *shiatsu* therapy from other healing models and massage therapies. When Western massage was introduced to Japan in the late 1880s, the many vocational schools that taught *anma* were dominated by blind instructors. However, this very limitation obstructed the further development of *anma* and led to the evolution of what we recognize today as *shiatsu* therapy.

Modern *shiatsu* is a product of twentieth-century refinements and evolution that produced the form of therapy used today. *Shiatsu* began its modern evolution in the 1920s (the Taisho period) when *anma* practitioners adopted some of the West's hands-on techniques, including those of chiropractic and physiotherapy.

The practice of *shiatsu* received support from studies conducted after World War II when U.S. Military Governor General Douglas McArthur directed the Japanese Health Ministry. There were more than 300 unregulated therapies in Japan at that time. McArthur ordered all 300 to be researched by scientists at the universities, to document which ones had scientific proof of merit, and which did not. At the end of eight years, the universities reported back that "shiatsu" was the only therapeutic practice to receive scientific approval at that time (Saito 2001).

In 1955 the Japanese parliament adopted a bill on "revised *anma*," which gave *shiatsu* official government endorsement. This endorsement allowed *shiatsu* to be legally taught in schools throughout Japan. *Shiatsu* received further official Japanese government recognition as a therapy in 1964. In the early 1970s *shiatsu* began spreading to the West and rapidly gained widespread acceptance (Cowmeadow 1992).

Although *shiatsu* and its distant cousin acupuncture are considered medically sound and are accepted methods of treatment for over one-quarter of the world's population, the United States and many other Western nations still consider both techniques experimental. However, several U.S. hospitals now allow the use of acupuncture, and medical students are taught the theories and practice of acupuncture, *shiatsu*, and macrobiotics. *Shiatsu* is part of the growing trend and movement toward integrative medicine.

Everything is energy

Many followers of Eastern traditions believe that the natural state of humanity is to be healthy. The simple understanding that humans are equipped to heal themselves, and that they can also help to heal others, forms the underlying foundation of *shiatsu*. *Shiatsu* acts like a spark or catalyst to the self-healing power of the human body, and a combination of treatment and healthy lifestyle form the basis of total care. The major underlying principle of *shiatsu*, derived from the tenets of Asian medicine, is actually a reflection of modern scientific thought.

Simply stated, "Everything is energy." When considered in the context of molecular structure, all matter is a manifestation of energy. *Shiatsu* interacts directly with this energy, and therefore with life itself.

From the perspective of classical Chinese medicine, energy moves along distinct pathways, meridians or channels (*kieraku* in Japanese). Accounts in the *shiatsu* tradition posit that meridians were discovered when certain acupoints (specific locations along the meridians) were stimulated and beneficial results were observed; for example, asthma-like symptoms caused by certain types of battle wounds were relieved when the corresponding acupoint was touched, and menstrual pain was reduced when a heated stone from a fireplace brushed against a point on the inner thigh.

Many studies have been conducted by biophysicists in Japan, China, and France. They postulate that a measurement of acupoint electricity provides a biophysical marker that illustrates the objective existence of the meridian system. They discovered that acupoints have a lower skin resistance. When an electrical current is passed through a classical acupoint, it has a higher electrical conductance, which is a lower resistance, than the surrounding area. They also discovered that when disease or illness is present, pathological changes take place in the body, and simultaneously changes are found in the resistance of relevant meridians and acupoints. Researchers also found that environmental factors such as temperature, season, and time of day, changed the resistance of acupoints.

In the Lanzhou Medical College in China a test of the acupoints of the stomach meridian showed significant variations in conductance when the stomach lining was stimulated by cold or hot water, either before or after eating (Yamamoto and McCarty 1993).

In addition to scientific evidence, the benefits of *shiatsu* are supported by the experiences of clients and practitioners alike. Asthmatic clients experience volatility (pain and sensitivity) along their lung meridian. Clients with lower digestive tract symptoms, such as constipation, experience this same sensitivity along their large intestine meridian.

Along the meridian lines are points called *tsubos* (pronounced "sue-bows"). The word *tsubo* is derived from the Chinese characters meaning "hole or orifice," and "position" (the position of the hole). Traditionally, the word "hole" was combined with other terms such as "hollow," "passageway," "transport," and *ki* (or vital energy). This suggests that the holes on the surface of the body were regarded as routes of access to the body's internal cavities. The acupoints are spots where it is accessed (Yamamoto and McCarty 1993).

Shiatsu sees three phases in the historical development of the concept of these holes or acupoints. In the earliest phase people would use any body location that was painful or uncomfortable. Because there were no specific locations for the points, they had no names. In the second phase, after a long period of practice and experience, certain points became identified with specific diseases. The ability of distinct points to affect and be affected by local or distant pain and disease became predictable. In the final phase, many previously localized points, each with a singular function, became integrated into a larger system that related and grouped diverse points systematically according to similar functions. This integration is called the meridian or channel system.

Although the analogy is not entirely accurate, *shiatsu* is often called "acupuncture without needles." To alter a client's internal energy system or pattern, an acupuncturist inserts needles into the *tsubos* used by a *shiatsu* practitioner. The most significant difference between the two disciplines is that acupuncture is invasive and is performed by extensively trained doctors, while *shiatsu* is noninvasive and can be practiced by either a professional therapist or a lay person. *Shiatsu* is also a whole-body technique, in contrast to one that is limited to the insertion of needles at specific *tsubos*. Acupuncture is considered more symptom-oriented, in that people are unlikely to go to an acupuncturist without a specific complaint, whereas clients often equate *shiatsu* with health maintenance and go for treatments without particular "problems." Although some consider *shiatsu* a cousin to acupuncture, others suggest a "distant cousin" relationship.

It is also important to note here that simple *shiatsu* can be practiced with little or no understanding of the underlying principles. The practitioner does not have to agree with the principles or understand them in order to provide *shiatsu*; however, the techniques are part of a more complicated healing system that, when adhered to and studied, provides more effective results (Palanjian 2002, p.144).

A simple and accurate analogy for understanding the meridian pathways and *tsubos* in relation to the body's internal organ systems is that *tsubos* can be compared to a system of volcanoes on the earth's surface. We know that a volcano's real energy is not at the surface, but is found deep inside the earth. A volcano is a superficial manifestation of the underlying energy. In similar fashion, a *tsubo* can be thought of as a manifestation of the underlying energy of the organ system. This does not imply that the therapist should ignore the area of pain that a *shiatsu* client may describe. However, a classically trained *shiatsu* practitioner looks beyond sore shoulders, ligaments, and tendons (unless the cause of the pain is trauma to these structures), and focuses on the related organ system via the meridian network. Philosophically, *shiatsu* practitioners relate health to the condition of the related "vital" organs (i.e. those associated with the meridian system). Although *shiatsu* is noninvasive and appears to deal with external or surface pain, according to *shiatsu* theory, it stimulates, sedates, and balances energy inside the body to address the root causes of surface and bodily discomfort (Palanjian 2002, p.145).

The principles of Asian medicine evident in *shiatsu* theory and practice maintain that two states exist in the universe. These two states, called yin and yang, exist side by side and are considered both complementary and opposing (see Chapter 3). Asian medicine looks at health more as a manifestation of balance between yin and yang, and in terms of how an imbalance may allow infection or disease to manifest. When a person's health and metabolism adjust to universal cosmic guidelines, natural harmony occurs from the inside out. Varying states of yin and yang are experienced.

In defining yin and yang, bear in mind that a continuum exists between the extremes of each. In *shiatsu*, major organs are *paired together* under one of the *five major elements*. Each pair has both a yang and a yin organ. One organ is more compact and tighter (yang), whereas the other is more open and vessel-like (yin) (see Chapter 3). The five elements, Wood (Tree), Fire, Earth (Soil), Metal, and Water, proceed clockwise around the five-element wheel used in Asian medicine. According to *shiatsu* principles, an organ is fed by its opposite energy (Palanjian 2002, p.145).

A yang organ is fed by yin energy and vice versa. A *shiatsu* practitioner generally describes the kidney as yang because of its compact structure, compared with its paired, more hollow and open yin organ, the bladder. Whereas *shiatsu* texts often use the term "structure" to describe an organ, acupuncture texts may describe the same organ in terms of the energy that feeds it through the meridian. A classically trained acupuncturist generally describes the kidney as yin because it is fed by yin energy that flows up the body on the Kidney meridian.

Such differences in descriptive language between the two disciplines can be confusing, although little if any differences in application of goals, practice, or theory really exists (Palanjian 2002, p.146).

Another major principle in *shiatsu* involves the concepts of *kyo* (pronounced "key-o") and *jitsu* ("jit-sue"). *Kyo* is considered empty or vacant, whereas *jitsu* is considered full, excessive, or overflowing. A *jitsu* condition along the Gallbladder meridian may be a manifestation of a gallbladder imbalance, resulting perhaps from recent consumption of a large pizza and two dishes of ice cream. A *kyo*, or empty, condition along the Lung meridian (and within the lung itself) may exist in an individual who doesn't exercise and rarely expands his or her chest cavity or heart.

Understanding and finding these energy manifestations is critical to diagnosis in *shiatsu* practice and is an ongoing, lifelong learning experience for the serious *shiatsu* practitioner. Although it is generally easy to find *jitsu*, or excess, it is much harder to find emptiness or vacancy (*kyo*) within the meridian network. One of the keys to doing highly successful or refined *shiatsu* is the ability to find specific *kyo* within the body or the organ's meridian network, and then to manipulate it effectively.

Shiatsu massage is not viewed by its practitioners as a panacea. *Shiatsu* philosophy is very clear in reinforcing the need for dietary and lifestyle guidance and changes to complement and support a *shiatsu* session (or series of sessions). The choices made by the recipients of treatment are theirs (Palanjian 2002, p.147). Many recipients are content to stay at the level at which *shiatsu* is simply used for pain reduction and for producing a "calmed sense of revitalization." However, others who are open to the underpinnings of *shiatsu* philosophy may be willing to take additional steps suggested by a classically trained *shiatsu* practitioner regarding diet and behavior modification.

With sufficient training, the *shiatsu* practitioner learns to view the energy manifesting at major *tsubos* on the surface of the skin as indicative of the underlying condition of the organs to which the *tsubos* are related and connected. For instance, a client may think shoulder pain is caused by how he or she sleeps, or sits at a desk. A classically trained *shiatsu* practitioner does not ignore these factors, but looks beyond to the underlying organ system and considers the foods that affect that organ system. The practitioner attempts to change the energy pattern, by working not just at the proximate points of client complaint and distress, but also along the entire related meridian (or set of meridians).

Shiatsu training touches on the principles of Asian medicine because the nature of the organ systems and their related energy should be understood for effective treatment to occur— although, as mentioned previously, this knowledge is not an absolute requirement to practice *shiatsu*. How far this education goes, particularly in relation to the underlying effects of specific foods and their yin and yang effects on various organs and the body as a whole, depends on the quality of the school, the knowledge of the instructor, and the interest of the students.

The art of diagnosis

The art of *shiatsu* diagnosis is a lifelong learning process. Subtle yet specific, diagnosis is an ongoing and evolving pursuit, in which a practitioner is continually mastering and learning. Modern diagnostic techniques are a relatively recent development in the history of medicine. Powerful, precise, and accurate to a large extent, their contribution to the improvement of the human condition cannot be denied. However, diagnostic procedures in Western medicine use a disease-oriented model and tend to focus on parts (e.g. cells, tissues, organs) rather than on the whole organism. For example, Louis Pasteur (1822–1895) believed that microbes were the primary cause of disease. Although this theory has proved correct and is applicable to a large number of cases, germs are not the sole cause of disease.

In *shiatsu*, there are two underlying levels of diagnosing human beings: *constitutional* and *conditional*. Simply stated, an individual's *constitution* is what he or she was born with. Along with inherited traits, the quality of life, energy, and food intake experienced by the mother while the baby is *in utero* are all considered factors that make up a person's constitution. A person's *condition* is the sum of his or her experience, which includes diet. In classical *shiatsu* diagnosis, both constitution and condition are assessed according to the following four methods of observing "phenomena":

1. *Bo-shin*: diagnosis through observation.

2. *Bun-shin*: diagnosis through sound.

3. *Mon-shin*: diagnosis through questioning.

4. *Set su-shin*: diagnosis through touch.

Each day, whether we realize it or not, we use the first three methods of observation extensively in our interactions with others and the environment. We have all experienced a funny feeling in the stomach when we enter a room that has recently been the site of some tense human interaction. We choose partners based on some innate recognition of energy we find compatible with our own. Although we are unaware that we are using aspects of Asian diagnosis in our everyday lives, we nonetheless make assessments and judgments based on these principles. Without these "diagnostic skills" we would not long survive. *Shiatsu* uses the first three methods liberally, and also relies heavily on the fourth (Palanjian 2002, p.148).

In traditional *shiatsu*, diagnosis begins with the first contact between client and practitioner, whether in person or on the telephone. The client's tone of voice, speed of delivery, and choice of words give clues to the trained ear regarding the condition and constitution of the client. On meeting a client for the first time, constitutional and conditional assessments are made. How did the client enter the room? Did she walk upright? Did he smile or frown? Was her handshake strong or weak? Was his hand wet, damp, dry, hot, cold? The client is often unaware that a classically trained *shiatsu* therapist begins work with the first contact and continues the assessment the minute a face-to-face meeting begins. Visual diagnosis and verbal questioning continue as the first meeting between client and therapist proceeds.

To arrive at a *constitutional* diagnosis, the therapist looks at various physical attributes. No single factor observed gives a total picture, but a macro-assessment takes the various micro-elements into account. Size of ears, shape and size of head, distance between the eyes, size of mouth, and size of hands are fundamental observations made in constitutional diagnosis before any physical treatment begins.

Factors considered in *conditional* assessment are slightly different but work in tandem with the overall assessment. The stated reason for the visit is a factor. In addition, tone and volume of the client's voice, pupil size, eye color, color and condition of the tongue, condition of the nails, and response to palpation along specific points on the hands and arms may be used. Pulse diagnosis (reading distinctly differently levels of heartbeats near the wrists on both hands) may be used, depending on the practitioner's level of training. Generally speaking, pulse diagnosis is more the tool of an acupuncturist, but it has been and can be used by a properly trained *shiatsu* provider.

These four diagnostic methods (observation, sound, questioning, and touch) are used to develop a singular yin–yang analysis. At its basic level, Asian diagnosis sets out to determine whether a person is vibrationally, or energetically, more yin or more yang, because these two opposing but complementary states of energy affect each of us.

The diagnostic assessment process continues along specific lines:

- *Yang diagnosis*: excess body heat and desire for coolness; great thirst and desire for fluids; constipation and hard stools; scanty, hot, dark urine.

- *Yin diagnosis*: cold feeling and desire for warmth; lack of thirst and preference for hot drinks; loose stools; profuse, clear urine; flat taste in mouth; poor appetite.

(Yamamoto and McCarty 1993)

The key is first, determining what tendency within an individual may be contributing to his or her state, and also the particular organ or organs that have a *jitsu* or *kyo* condition, and then working those organs' meridians to change that state.

At this point, the practitioner's hands become the primary diagnostic tools. Although diagnosis is an ongoing process during treatment, traditional *shiatsu* may first assess by palpation the major organs located in the client's *hara*, or abdomen. Alternatively, some styles of *shiatsu* begin a treatment session with touch diagnosis on the upper back, an area that also yields a vast amount of information regarding a person's condition. Assessment and diagnosis include palpatory observations that describe the following physical properties: tightness or looseness, fullness or emptiness, hot or cold, dry or wet, resistant or open, stiff or flexible.

Diagnosis in a *shiatsu* session does not cease after an initial assessment but is an ongoing process of observation, listening, feeling, and changing focus, based on continuously revealed information. The ability to make a quick, accurate diagnosis can be extremely helpful to both the practitioner and the client in their mutual attempt to create energetic change for the receiving partner. However, *shiatsu* can be effective in the hands of a relatively unskilled diagnostician. By following the simple principle of paying attention to what is going on under one's hands, a lay person, with relatively little training, can provide an effective, relaxing, and enjoyable *shiatsu* treatment for family and friends in a nonprofessional setting (Palanjian 2002, p.149).

Learning shiatsu

Unlike some disciplines, *shiatsu* is easy to learn. It is not possible for a lay person to practice chiropractic, acupuncture, or osteopathy, because medical professionals need not only training but also time and continuing education to master techniques and improve skills. *Shiatsu* also requires a disciplined approach, constant practice, and continuing study to develop in-depth understanding. However, the practice remains simple, effective, and safe. *Shiatsu* techniques can be learned and safely applied by anyone, typically resulting in positive effects for both the recipient and the provider. It can be performed anywhere, takes place with the client fully clothed, and requires no special tools, machines, or oils (Sergel 1989).

While *ki* does indeed emanate from the giver's fingertips, it may not be in this way or only in this way that *shiatsu* works. Indeed, *shiatsu* training often emphasizes that the most important element is to be in touch with what is going on *right under one's hands*. Experts agree, indicating that when a practitioner applies pressure and stimulation, he or she should then react and follow up based on an intuitive sense of, and response to, internal changes within the recipient. A traditionally trained *shiatsu* practitioner, knowledgeable in the energy fundamentals of yin and yang and applying those principles in his or her life, is arguably better able to respond intuitively to the client. It is believed that intuition is enhanced by being in harmony with nature, a condition achieved by following the guidelines of living within nature's principles and the earth's rhythms of yin and yang. Harmony in the body is achieved by being in harmony with the universe.

Relaxed and revitalized

Because *shiatsu* can yield a "calmed sense of revitalization," the combination of being both *relaxed and energized* is an experience that may be savored throughout the day. Americans often equate "calm and relaxed" with an inactive state. Although *shiatsu* yields different results for different people, one of the most unique effects experienced by most clients is indeed this "calmed sense of revitalization." It is not uncommon for a new *shiatsu* client to report, when treated by a competent practitioner, that he or she has "never felt this way before" (Palanjian 2002, p.149).

One reason for the difference in the energetic effects of *shiatsu* as distinct from other techniques (usually called regular massage by the general public) is easy to explain. In many forms of therapeutic massage a technique described as *effleurage* or stroking (sweeping the skin with the hands) is used. The benefits of this type of movement on the skin are many, including stimulation of blood flow and the movement of lymph. Although this technique is beneficial, one of its effects is often a feeling of lethargy. Because the effects of *shiatsu* are realized more on the underlying blockage of energy related to the body's organ systems than on the lymphatic system, a *shiatsu* session can yield a feeling of increased short- and long-term energy. This is why chair massage using *shiatsu* techniques is so appropriate, and considered by many superior to other techniques in the corporate setting. Employees do not experience the short-term negative energetic effects (lethargy) of *effleurage*, but rather the energetic boost, the *calmed sense of revitalization* so often associated with effective *shiatsu* technique.

Both *anma* and European massage directly stimulate blood circulation, emphasizing the release of stagnated blood in the skin and muscles together with tension and stiffness resulting from circulatory congestion. On the other hand, *shiatsu* emphasizes correction and maintenance of bone structure, joints, tendons, muscles, and meridian lines whose malfunctioning distort the body's energy and autonomic nervous system, causing disease (Masunaga and Oshashi 1977).

Like other methods, *shiatsu* is best received with an empty stomach. This may not always be possible, and recent food consumption is certainly no bar to receiving *shiatsu*. However, practitioners and recipients should bear in mind that when the body's energies are focused inward toward digestion, a *shiatsu* session, with its attempt to change the body's energies, is compromised and less effective.

In some ways the beginning of a *shiatsu* session is similar to other massage styles. The room used should be simple, clean, and quiet. A thorough history of the client and his or her concerns should be taken. Questions regarding sleep patterns, lifestyle, eating habits, and work history are not uncommon. A high level of trust should be established quickly. Often a client is seated in a chair or on a floor mat, as the *shiatsu* practitioner observes and asks questions regarding the client's expectations and level of understanding. Diagnostic techniques to determine the client's constitution and condition are undertaken. The hands, eyes, tongue, and coloration along the upper and lower limbs may be examined. Several deep breaths to begin the process may be suggested. A well-trained *shiatsu* practitioner obtains a complete history to uncover any risk factors affecting the appropriateness of *shiatsu* treatment. Clinical experience and training, coupled with good references regarding a therapist's skills and practice, should be the determining factors in selecting a *shiatsu* practitioner. There are many variations on the basic techniques, and numerous schools that teach specific *shiatsu* practices offer more distinct focus on the underlying themes outlined above. The American Organization for Bodywork Therapies of Asia (AOBTA) notes 12 specific areas of Asian technique. The major schools of Asian practice generally regarded as *shiatsu* are described in the following sections (AOBTA 2001; see also the AOBTA website, www.aobta.org).

Five element shiatsu

The primary emphasis of five element *shiatsu* is to identify a pattern of disharmony by means of the four examinations, and to harmonize that pattern with an appropriate treatment plan. Hands-on techniques and preferences for assessment vary with the practitioner, depending on individual background and training. The radial pulse usually provides the most critical and detailed information. Palpation of the back and/or abdomen and a detailed verbal history serve to confirm the assessment. Considerations of the client's lifestyle, emotional, and psychological factors are all considered important. Although this approach uses the paradigm of the five elements to tonify, sedate or control patterns of disharmony, practitioners of this style also consider hot or cold, internal, or external symptoms and signs (Palanjian 2002, p.153).

Japanese shiatsu

Although *shiatsu* is primarily the application of pressure, usually with the thumbs along the meridian lines, extensive soft tissue manipulation and both active and passive exercise and stretching may be part of the treatments. Extensive use of cutaneous-visceral reflexes in the abdomen and on the back are also characteristics of *shiatsu*. The emphasis of *shiatsu* is the treatment of the whole meridian; however, effective points are also used. The therapist assesses the condition of the patient's body as treatment progresses. Therapy and diagnosis are one.

Macrobiotic shiatsu

Founded by Shizuko Yamamoto and based on George Ohsawa's philosophy that each individual is an integral part of nature (see Chapter 9), macrobiotic *shiatsu* supports a natural lifestyle and heightened instincts for improving health. Assessments are through visual, verbal, and touch techniques (including pulses).

Treatment involves noninvasive touch and pressure using hand and barefoot techniques and stretches to facilitate the flow of *ki* and to strengthen the body–mind. Dietary guidance, medicinal plant foods, breathing techniques and home remedies are emphasized, and corrective exercises, postural rebalancing, palm healing, self *shiatsu,* and *qi gong* are included in macrobiotic *shiatsu.*

Shiatsu anma therapy

Shiatsu anma therapy utilizes a unique blending of two of the most popular Asian bodywork forms practiced in Japan, *shiatsu* and *anma* massage.

Zen shiatsu

Zen *shiatsu* is characterized by the theory of *kyo–jitsu* (see page 116 above), its physical and psychological manifestations, and its application to abdominal diagnosis. Zen *shiatsu* theory is based on an extended meridian system that includes as well as expands the location of the traditional acupuncture meridians. The focus of a Zen *shiatsu* session is on the use of meridian lines rather than on specific points. In addition, Zen *shiatsu* does not adhere to a fixed sequence or set of methods that are applied to all. It utilizes appropriate methods for the unique pattern of each individual (AOBTA 2001).

Finding a practitioner

As of July 2011, there are currently no government regulatory standards in the United States for *shiatsu* practitioners, whereas MassageMag.com notes that 42 states, the District of Columbia, and four Canadian provinces currently offer some type of credential to professionals in the massage or bodywork field— usually licensure, certification, or registration. There are over 300,000 certified practitioners at the time of writing. Numerous schools of massage offer certificate programs in *shiatsu*, or more broad-based programs that include *shiatsu* massage. These programs may be weekend seminars of one or two days, or may provide 600 or more hours of training particular to *shiatsu*. It is not uncommon for schools to offer 350 to 500 hours of training in classical *shiatsu*, with an additional 150 hours in anatomy and physiology. There appears to be a growing trend for internships in all schools of massage.

The American Organization for Bodywork Therapies of Asia, (AOBTA, formerly the American Asian Body Therapy Association) is the largest and most widespread organization particular to the practice of *shiatsu*. Certified practitioner applicants must complete a 500-hour program, preferably at a school or institution recognized by AOBTA.

The American Massage Therapy Association (AMTA) is a general association of massage practitioners; it does not actively focus on *shiatsu* therapy. It is a highly respected association that meets with AOBTA as a federated massage-supporting organization. AMTA's mission is to develop and advance the art, science, and practice of massage therapy in a caring, professional, and ethical manner to promote the health and welfare of humanity.

The American Bodywork and Massage Professionals (ABMP) is another highly respected association of massage professionals. Unlike AOBTA and AMTA, ABMP is a for-profit organization.

The National Certification Board for Therapeutic Massage and Bodywork (NCBTMB) is a nationally recognized certifying body formed to set high standards for those who practice therapeutic massage and bodywork. It accomplishes this through a nationally recognized certification program that assesses the competence of its practitioners. As of July 2011, close to 100,000 massage therapists and bodyworkers have received certification since 1992. The NCBTMB examination is now legally recognized in most states and in many municipalities. The NCBTMB represents a diverse group of massage therapists, not only *shiatsu* practitioners. A minimum of 500 hours of formal massage education and successful completion of a written exam are the basic requirements for certification. Practitioners must be re-certified every four years (Palanjian 2002, p.153).

A person considering the use of any massage therapy as an adjunct to health maintenance should carefully select the provider of that therapy. In addition to personal references, it is important to evaluate the practitioner's training, experience, professional affiliations, and certification.

The concluding pages of Part II provide good guidance for using all the treatments that have been presented in Parts I and II and that are available in Europe and the United States.

The Southeast Asian healing traditions we will encounter in Part III demonstrate the influence of Greater Chinese medical concepts but, unlike Chinese medicine, they are not organized as complete and complex, national, regional, or global medical health care systems, nor are they available on any regular basis in Europe and North America. Nonetheless, they offer effective herbal remedies which are available to us worldwide, dating back to the historic European mercantile trade, and later the U.S. "China and Japan Trade," with the legendary Spice Islands (see Appendix II). They also offer important lessons in the role of celestial wisdom, divine spirit, natural order, and community cohesion in effecting health and healing for all peoples.

PART III

❧

Southeast Asia

Chapter 11

The Celestial and
the Shamanic

Shamanic Chinese medicine

In prehistoric times, Chinese medicine was not yet concerned with channeling revealed heavenly knowledge from celestial sources for health and healing, but rather with battling demonic forces that caused illness and disease. (See "Chronological Phases of Chinese Medicine" table on p.viii.) This primordial battle against disease-causing demons pre-dated developments in Chinese medical theory that would later seek balance and harmony within the individual; in fact, the sick individual was not "treated" at all. Rather, magicians and healers directed their attentions and efforts only to placating the dead ancestors and demons that determined fate. The "patient" was never examined or touched at all in this kind of "healing."

Prehistoric Chinese medicine was essentially shamanism—the kind of traditional healing that the organized, systematic, celestial healing of Chinese medical treatment proper, derived from the three divine emperors, would later encounter in Southeast Asia during the era of the expansion of Greater China.

In fact, in our Western view, the concept and the very term *shamanism* originated in application to traditional spirit healers, or medicine men, of North Central Asia—what is today Siberia in Russia, Manchuria in China, and the northern Korean Peninsula—possibly holdovers from the prehistoric type of Chinese medicine men that held sway before the advent of modern, naturalistic concepts of health and healing.

In this way, Chinese medicine itself started as "shamanic" healing, with oracle bones and diviners, and demon-exorcising *wu* (*magician-healers*). Later, having become a more organized, theoretically sophisticated and systematic form of medicine, it again encountered shamanic healing traditions in Southeast Asia during the era of Greater China—and grafted its more organized views on the celestial origins of medical knowledge and practice onto the "primitive" practices of demon-haunted Southeast Asia.

Taking the word *shaman* out of cold storage

"Shaman" is a word that comes from the *Tungus* language of Central Siberia. The term incorporates men and women as religious leaders who serve their community by use of drums to call spirit allies. It is a priestly vocation and cannot typically be "learned," as most shamans are born to such a calling. It is important to note this definition as a fundamental point because the word has drawn many different, false definitions, and people have misused it.

The original term "shamanism" has now taken on a meaning in the wider academic world as well as in popular culture. It recognizes that indigenous societies have "spiritual" practitioners outside the confines of recognized, organized "religions." While its origin lies in a specific definition relating to societies in Central Siberia and Manchuria, the general usage of the term fulfills the need to describe a widespread cultural phenomenon among indigenous peoples in traditional societies worldwide, beyond the confines of Siberia, Manchuria, and ancient China.

Table 11.1 Views of sickness and healing related to the stages of human social evolution*

Social type	Subsistence	Causation of illness	Healers
Nomadic	Hunter-gatherer foraging	Self, ancestors, deity, "outsiders"	Shamans, diviners
Village	Simple horticulture	Commnity members, simple ethno-pathology	Shamans, magico-religious healers, spiritual mediums, herbalists
Nomadic pastoralists	Herding, animal domestication	Imbalances in hot and cold	Healers, spiritual mediums, exorcists
Chiefdoms	Sedentary agriculture	Imbalances in "humors"	Healers, spiritual mediums, herbalists, shamans
Early states	Complex agriculture	Imbalances	Same as above, plus priests
Civilizations	Irrigation agriculture	Individual behavior, moral failings, imbalances, elaborate ethnopath-ology	Priests, physicians, folk and religious healers
Modern industrial	Mechanized	Germs, genes, lifestyles, elaborate pathologies	Physicians, folk healers, alternative practitioners
Postmodern	Information	Mind–body imbalances "humors"	Integration

*Adapted from Horatio Fabrega, Jr. (1997) *Evolution of Healing and Sickness*. Berkeley: University of California.

There is evidence reflecting concern with human illness and disease in ancient China dating back to 1500 BCE. The first 1000 years of general archaeological evidence, prior to the origin, or restrospective compilation, of classic Chinese medical texts, reflects concerns with oracular therapy, demonic medicine, and religious healing. Eventually, with the development of Chinese medicine proper, the demons would be exorcised and banished to the far reaches of the Malay Peninsula, Indonesian Archipelago, and Philippine Islands, where they would flourish through their later encounter with the official medicine, of Greater China.

In prehistoric China, illness and disease were believed to be caused by supernatural phenomena, rather than by natural causes—that is by ancestors, spirits and demons, gods, and transcendental law. These associations reflect general observations about disease and medicine as related to the stages of evolution in human society, as shown in Table 11.1.

The Shang and the Ancestors

The civilization of the Shang arose along the middle course of the Yellow River (in modern Hunan Province) in the period from 1800–1600 BCE. Information about this period is drawn largely from archaeology, although there was a written language using some of the Chinese pictographs that are still in use today.

A great number of inscribed bones and tortoiseshells— "oracle bones"—from this era have been recovered over the past century. Although the great mass of people still lived with Stone Age technology, metallurgy was advanced into the Bronze and Iron Ages. The origin and purpose of a number of large cast bronze vessels dating from the sixteenth to second century BCE used in court and burial rituals have remained a mystery to experts on ancient Chinese civilization—but the author of this book has long proposed the idea that these pots were used for boiling animal carcasses for the purpose of deriving oracle bones, and represented the best available method of so doing. The bones, initially of cattle, later of tortoises, were used to communicate with the ancestors. Heating the bones would cause cracks to appear that could then be interpreted as signaling the answers and intentions of the ancestors.

When it came to illness and disease, pathophysiological phenomena were observed and systematically labeled as "blow of a demon" (heart attack), or the more versatile "curse of an ancestor," which covered toothache, headache, abdominal distention, or leg pains. The ultimate balance to be achieved for the avoidance of illness and disease was harmony between the living and the ancestors. The notion of balance within the individual, or between the individual and Nature, would come later.

The Shang also believed in other causes of illness, about which the ancestors nonetheless understood, such as "malignant wind" from wind-spirits. According to bone inscriptions the *wu* (ancient Chinese shaman) could control the forces of the wind. Evil wind may have acted in its own right, or may have been used as a tool by evil ancestors. The theme of wind sickness is widespread throughout modern Southeast Asia. The desire to this day among Chinese communities in Hong Kong and Taiwan, for example, to have their ancestors' bones passed over by good "wind and water" (modern *feng-shui*) in their burial grounds is an echo of the ancient winds of the Shang.

Finally, Shang oracle bones sometimes showed a character (subsequently used from the Han Period onward) for "black magic," that is, deliberate illness-causing intentions of one person against another.

The interventions of *wu* shamans with the ancestors did not directly involve any real contact with the "patient." Healers who dealt with the actual physical aspect of the sick individual did not yet appear in favor of the purely "social therapy" conducted by the *wu*. This social therapy has strong parallels in the communal healing rituals found throughout Southeast Asia.

The warring of states and the releasing of demons

The Shang Dynasty gave way to the Zhou, a semi-nomadic group from the northwest who settled down to develop communally managed irrigation agriculture, which granted them an advantage. The Zhou Dynasty manifests certain political parallels to the era of feudalism in Europe. There was a long period of bloody strife, giving way to what is known as the "Warring States" period throughout much of China. Ultimately the Qin Dynasty was able to subdue all rivals in the third century BCE, by effectively rejecting what might be called the code of "chivalry" in favor of "total war." Finally these excesses led to eradication of the Qin by 200 BCE in favor of the Han Dynasty, whose fourth emperor, Wu, brought China a period of peace and stability and a social-political system that was to be characteristic for the next 2000 years.

Given the violent excess of the Zhou and Qin dynasties it is not surprising that during the Zhou period demons had been loosed upon the living and came to be seen as responsible for everyday misfortunes, including illness, diminishing the role of ancestors. The *wu* of the Shang period were adopted as leaders who were believed to possess magical powers. The pictograph for *wu* has a dancing figure at its core—a primary function and method of "medicine men" and shamans worldwide. With the temporary break-down of the old system of the earth and the ancestors, rifts opened between the realms of the living and the dead, creating myths about the role of demons in exerting influences over the living. Exorcism became the chief responsibility of the *wu*. The ancestors had lost control over their living descendants, whose fates were cast into the hands of demons that could freely roam from one person to another. In contrast to both the prior Ancestor medicine, and the Confucian system then being born, the cause of disease during the "Warring States" period may best be described as "all against all." Typical demonic illnesses were labeled as "assaulted by demons," "possessed by the hostile (influences of demonic guests)," and "struck by evil."

The efforts of the *wu* were directed to expelling demons, often by thrusting spears into the air or, more dramatically, into unfortunate political prisoners. The Chinese character used for "healing" and "healer" shows the dancing character for *wu* in the lower half, and an arrow in a quiver, and a lance or spear, in the upper half. *Breath magic*, including blowing, spitting and shouting, was believed to be like blowing out the stream of fire to the spiritual world. Such procedures are also used by shamans worldwide.

Rhythmic banging on drums, gongs or chimes, shouting and chanting, was another means to drive away demons. Likewise, burning of talismans transported the written word to a spiritual destination. The entire population also wore talismans of wood, jade or gold, depending upon the means of the wearer. *Wu* exorcists prepared talismans in the form of official state documents which would "command" demons to leave. These may have been the first prescriptions. Incantations had the same purpose.

Of interest is the manipulation of what are believed to have been acupuncture points—at that time labeled "demon camp," "demon heart," "demon path," "demon bed," and "demon hall." The needles used to penetrate "demon heart" were analogous to the spears used by exorcists. Although there is no written reference to therapeutic acupuncture needling prior to the first century BCE, the possibility that acupuncture originally, under the Han, had a purely demonic medicine function can not be ruled out; the long persistence of many of these practices may ultimately be better explained in terms of their resonance with *battling* social and political developments in ancient China, than by their consistency with later *balancing* Buddhist and Daoist philosophies.

Ultimately, as time passed, spiritual powers began to be seen as emanating from celestial sources (characteristic of later Chinese civilization) and the *chu* (*priests* or *supplicants*) supplanted the supernatural demon practitioners. The *chu* no longer held spiritual powers themselves, as the *wu* had, but simply tried to access the divine sources of power, which ultimately were associated with the semi-mythical emperors and their brethren. As for the demons, they sought the warmer climes of Southeast Asia, where a shamanic system of traditional healing persisted long after the development of Chinese medicine proper.

Chapter 12

Traditional Medicines of Southeast Asia

Cultural and Natural Influences

Southeast Asia and Greater China

Concepts of energy, mind and spirit which appear common to all traditional medicines are evident with the spread of Chinese influences, and their encounter with indigenous healing, throughout Southeast Asia. When considering the medical traditions of Southeast Asia, it is useful to recognize that almost all these territories came under the influence of two of the earliest civilizations at the dawn of history. The cultural diffusion first, of "Further India," and later of "Greater China," represented successive waves of influence emanating from the great river valleys of the Indus and the Yellow River respectively, carrying along common discoveries and understandings of the nature of human life and health.

The original center of Indian or Hindu culture and Sanskrit language texts was located in the Indus River Valley (modern-day Pakistan) in the second millennium BCE. Indo-European (or Aryan) peoples, originally from the Caucasus Mountains, had migrated east and south into the Indian subcontinent, establishing a new center in the Ganges River Valley at the foot of the Himalaya mountains, during the first millennium BCE, carrying Sanskrit texts and knowledge with them. This Hindu civilization, which we associate with Ayurvedic medicine and the related but separate practice of yoga, pushed the Dravidian peoples, whom we associate with Siddha medicine of South India, into the southeastern tip of India and onto the island of Ceylon, or Sri Lanka (see Micozzi 2011). One can see the subsequent outgrowth of Buddhism, originating from the Hindu Prince Siddhartha Gautama (the Buddha), as a second wave of influence from "Further India" giving birth to the new wave in Greater China, and East and Southeast Asia, including Indochina (today's Vietnam, Laos, and Cambodia). The very name "Indochina" implies this *overlap* of India and China.

Ultimately a third wave, Islam, spread during the seven hundred years 750–1450 CE, all the way to the western border of North Africa, and east through India and Malaya to the southern Philippines and the eastern edge of Indonesia. Islam also carried along Greek–Roman or Unani (the Arabic word for "Greek") concepts of health and healing, which it had incorporated and preserved following the ancient classical era in the West, and to which it added many important insights and practices. Bali, in the center of Indonesia, was "skipped over" by Islam, and retained its Indian Vedic roots; while Sri Lanka, off the far southeast coast of India, and Timor, at the far eastern edge of Indonesia, represent cultural fault lines which have had serious geopolitical repercussions right into the twenty-first century.

All three of these great successive traditions, Hindu-Vedic, Chinese, and Islamic–Unani, placed emphasis on the concept of vital energy, mind and spirit as central to health and healing.

In India, the geographic center of Asia, there were centuries of foreign rule, beginning in the fifteenth century when invaders from Persia (modern-day Iran) occupied neighboring parts of India, carrying the banner of Islam. They established the Mogul Empire, which was dominant especially in Northern India until the period of European colonization in Asia.

Hemispheres of influence

Initially, in the sixteenth century, the Portuguese established missions in South, Southeast, and East Asia under the dominions established by the Roman Catholic Pope Alexander VI in 1494 by the Treaty of Tordesillas at Valladolid, Spain. This decree divided the globe into two hemispheres along a line of longitude through the Atlantic Ocean (and on the other side of the globe through the Pacific) between the "eastern" half, under Portuguese influence, and the "western" half, under Spanish influence, for purposes of trade and evangelization.

The borders of these *"hemispheres of influence"* extended longitudinally around the globe. Eventually the Portuguese had an outpost in Brazil in the New World (at the western edge of the eastern hemisphere), while the Spanish developed a foothold in the Philippines in Asia (at the far western edge of the western hemisphere).

India, Malaya, and Indonesia (the "Spice Islands" of huge interest to the mercantile trade of that time) were firmly in the Portuguese half, as evidenced by the development of settlements extending from Goa at the western end, via Malacca on the Malay Peninsula in the middle to Timor at the eastern edge of Indonesia, in a vast sweep across Asia. All remain active settlements of Portuguese Roman Catholic life to this day.

The long-term influence of the Spanish in the Philippines led to the development of a syncretic brand of faith healing, intermingling Asian concepts of vital energy with Roman Catholic charismatic religious and spiritual practices. After the Spanish American War of 1898, and the 25-year effort by the United States to "pacify" the southern, Islamic, half of the Philippine Islands, there still remained many pockets of traditional Islamic and ethnomedical practices, which survived well into the second half of the twentieth century (see Chapter 14).

Going Dutch (and other Europeans)

During the seventeenth century, the dominance of Portugal and Spain in global trade and colonization slowly gave way to the Dutch in Malaya and Indonesia. The Dutch continued to focus their interests on the ancient territories of "Further India" in the

Indonesian archipelago, where Bali still survives as a remnant of ancient Hindu and Vedic civilization, amid a sea of subsequent influences from Islam.

Then, during the eighteenth century, influence passed to the French in India (Pondicherry) and Indochina (Vietnam), and to the English in India, Burma, and Malaya, with a foothold in the Chinese treaty port of Hong Kong. Ultimately European influence parceled itself out in such a way that, by the nineteenth century, India, Burma and Malaya were in the sphere of Great Britain, and Indochina (Vietnam) in the sphere of France, while Indonesia remained with the Dutch, and the Philippines with Spain (subject to occasional forays by the British). The Portuguese became relegated to their few remaining footholds in Goa, Macao, Malacca and Timor. The ancient Buddhist Kingdom of Siam (Thailand) always remained independent as a *de facto* buffer zone between Britain and France, its influence extending to the Lao people of Northwest Indochina (Laos).

The long independence of Thailand as a political state, with a divine, celestial ruler and strong Buddhist influences, as in ancient China, fostered a distinctive medical practice (see Chapter 15). The remnants of Indian influence are also preserved, as depicted in Thai representations and re-enactments of the Ramayana epic, for example. The celestial rulers of Thailand remain in place to this day, whereas the "Last Emperor" of China survived only the first decade of the twentieth century (except for the brief period of rule in *Manchukuo*, the Japanese puppet state in Northern China, or Manchuria, during World War II).

The role of energy, mind and spirit are central in all these medical traditions, which also share the belief that healing ultimately emanates from celestial or divine spiritual sources (as clearly articulated in the development of Chinese medicine itself). As we have discussed earlier in the book, Chinese medicine has its influence in Southeast Asia as a result of both (1) dissemination and diffusion of the concepts and theories of Chinese medicine, during particular historic periods, into indigenous medical traditions, and (2) the arrival of millions of "overseas Chinese" as immigrants during the eighteenth- and nineteenth-century era of European colonialism in Southeast

Asia, who in effect acted as emissaries, bringing Chinese medicine with them. In addition, as we have seen, Chinese migrants to new lands brought back new *materia medica* that were incorporated into Chinese medicine itself. More than anything it is this kind of exchange that characterizes the concept of "Greater China" with respect to medicine and other key aspects of social development within the Chinese sphere of influence.

The Malay Peninsula

A clear example is that of Malaysia (Malaya, prior to independence from Britain in 1962). In addition to indigenous Malay practices, there were early Indian and Chinese influences, followed by Islamic conversion, and later by successive waves of Europeans—Portuguese, Dutch and British. Further, under British control, Malaya saw the immigration of many Chinese, primarily to engage in local commerce and work in the rich tin mines, and also Indians, to work on the agricultural plantations of palm oil, rubber (once it arrived from the Amazon Basin), and coconut. Nineteenth-century migration witnessed the re-introduction of Indian and Chinese influences. Today, the population of Malaysia is approximately 60 percent Malay, 23 percent Chinese, and 7 percent Indian, with 10 percent of other ethnic origin. This rich mix supports the practice of many different medical traditions, side by side.

Throughout the Malay Peninsula and islands of Southeast Asia, there are also the *orang asli*, or "original men," in *Bahasa Malay*, who represent the indigenous peoples (probably related to the Aborigines of Australia). When the proto-Malaya subsequently arrived in ancient times throughout the region they pushed back these original inhabitants to where they can be found today: in the deep interior, high in the mountain regions (such as the Semang or "Negritos" in the center of Malaysia). The proto-Malay were supplanted in turn, by the Malay of today, who pushed them into the hinterlands where they are found today—for example, as the *Manobo*, *Tiboli*, and *Subanum* of the Southern Philippines (see Chapter 14), the "Montagnards" of Indochina, the interior tribes of Formosa

(Taiwan, or Nationalist China), and the "outer" islands of Japan, such as Okinawa in the south, and Hokaido in the north.

Each population has its own ethnomedical traditions, typically drawing from the concepts that are common to medical traditions in Greater China, as well as utilizing local indigenous *materia medica*. While there are cultural boundaries among healing traditions, there is also commonality among them.

Natural boundaries have also influenced ethnomedical traditions, as the following section describes.

Natural boundaries: the Wallace Line

Throughout this book we have illustrated how medical practices throughout Greater China are guided by the concepts of vital energy and celestial revelation, and are also influenced by the local *materia medica* as part of the ecology indigenous to each region. In addition to the historic political demarcation line between Portugal and Spain that ran through Southeast Asia from the sixteenth century onwards, there is also another important line of demarcation relating to the native *flora* and *fauna* (the basis of *materia medica*): the "Wallace Line" that runs generally north and south through the middle of the Southeast Asian Archipelago. Identified by the nineteenth century British natural scientist, Alfred Russel Wallace, this line traces the boundary between, on the one hand, the Asian, and on the other, the primarily Australian and Pacific ecological zones. Between the two lies the richest and most exotic assortment of terrestrial plants and animals anywhere on earth, including the legendary *Komodo dragon* and the *Bird of Paradise* (the bird itself, not the flower named after it), as well as unusual, highly nutritious fruits that cannot grow anywhere else on the planet (*durian, mangosteen, rambutan*). By studying this rich diversity, Wallace in fact came to understand the principles of natural selection and evolution long before Charles Darwin was able to formulate his own theory, based on observations that he had made on the Galapagos Islands during his much earlier voyage on *HMS Beagle*. It was Wallace who finally convinced Darwin to come forward with the theory of evolution, decades later.

Wallace also had the opportunity to observe and document many ethnomedical practices, as well as medicinal herbs and foods, throughout the *Malay Archipelago*, which he reported in his famous book of the same name, dedicated to Charles Darwin. Some of the medicinal herbs documented and recorded by Wallace are included in Appendix II.

Chapter 13

The Malay Peninsula and the Indonesian Archipelago

The most recent form of social organization in the Malay Peninsula prior to unification under the British Empire, and since gaining political independence in 1962, is a system of Islamic sultanates. These sultanates correspond approximately to the provinces or states of modern-day Malaysia. In addition to the Malay Peninsula, the former sultanates of Sabah and Sarawak, on the northwestern coast of the large island of Borneo to the east, also form part of Malaysia. (Borneo also contains the independent nation state of Brunei and the large Kalimantan province of Indonesia.)

Influences from Further India, Greater China and Islam have mixed with the ethnomedical practices of the indigenous Malay people. The sultanates of Kelantan and Tringganu on the eastern coast of Malaysia are considered as a seat of traditional Malay culture. Here it is generally acknowledged that Western health care can do little for diseases of the *spirit*, and that Western psychotherapy has little place; illnesses involving the spirit are a major category of disease, and care of the spirit is the province of shamans, called *bomoh*, or faith healers.

In the traditional healing of Southeast Asia, the concept of celestial origin of the knowledge of healing is evident, as in ancient China, and spiritual aspects of healing predominate. As in the ancient, prehistoric, more "primitive" aspects of Chinese medicine (preceding the advent of acupuncture, *tui na*, and *qi gong*) for the manipulation of vital energy (see Chapter 12), and Shintoism in Japan (see Chapter 10), traditional healing remains close to nature (see Chapter 12). Naturalistic origins of illness and paths to healing are therefore ascribed to observable natural phenomena, like the wind—literally, (as distinct from the more symbolic representation of Wind in five-elements Chinese medicine, for example). In fact, the idea that illness is carried "on the wind" has been compared by some Western observers to the idea of airborne pathogens (germs or microbes), which came to currency in Western thinking only in the late nineteenth century.

The traditional healer channels energies from celestial sources for both diagnostic and therapeutic purposes. Diagnoses and prescriptions in traditional medicine in Malaya are said to be "written on the wind," and the process of healing is likened to "taming the wind of desire."

Written on the wind

Three general types of illness are identified in traditional Malayan ethnomedicine. *Sakit biyasa* is ordinary sickness, and *sakit hangin* is, literally, sickness (*sakit*) from the wind or "moving air" (*hangin*). The third variety of illness is intermediate between these two and also attributes a large component of illness to spirit. More than just "catching a cold" in a draft (as in Western folklore), the wind imagery carries a literal meaning, in the sense that air rushing into the body is believed to result in disease. For example, in Malaysia and the Philippines (see Chapters 13 and 14), the most widely used traditional method of birth control, *coitus interruptus*, was believed to be detrimental to health, because when the penis is abruptly withdrawn air rushes into the womb, inflicting internal disturbances.

Aside from sexual desire, the wind imagery for sickness includes a symbolic "wind of desire" in the heart, whereby continual denial of emotion leads to illness. The Malay attitude "it is nothing only" (*walay lang*) in the face of emotionally charged events, and the striving to "save face" in public, produce a denial of feelings that may eventually take its toll, potentially leading either to *sakit hangin* (internalizing injuries), or literally running *amok* (itself a Malay word) and externalizing injuries by inflicting them on other parties.

Healers and healing rituals

Traditional Malay medicine is practiced by an estimated 2000 full-time and 20,000 part-time *bomoh* healers. Although *bomohs* share a number of characteristic skills, there is no single training path for these folk healers. Some have studied a few existing texts (mostly in Bahasa Malay of Javanese origin), but most learn from special teachers, usually their fathers, or gain special knowledge by revelation through dreams, waking encounters, or by inheriting a familiar, or helping spirit—a *hantu raya*.

Bomohs may be approximately categorized as spiritualists, herbalists, or traditional bonesetters, but there are no rigid specializations. Most *bomohs* use supernatural or Islamic incantations, but also know a great about herbal remedies for treating patients. Some also perform massages and special cleansing baths, and place "charms" on their patients. The *bomoh*'s *hantu raya*, in addition to helping heal, may also warn against returning to habits that cause bad health.

For a healing ritual, a *bomoh* involves the entire community. A *konduri*, or ritual communal meal, is offered with the performers of the healing. Communal meals of this kind are also held for courtships, contracts, or even car accidents today, as well as for healing. Symbolic foods such as *betel* nut and fish curry are prepared, and young coconuts are scored with spices and tobacco placed inside. The use of various indigenous *materia medica* draws on both the pharmacological properties of the constituents, such as betel nut, curry (coriander, cumin, turmeric), and tobacco (nicotine), and the symbolic significance of the ritual plants (equivalent to a "placebo" effect; Micozzi 1983).

Healing sounds in the rainforest

The *bomoh* goes into a trance in the company of a *mindok*—a partner, who does not, however, also go into trance. Instrumental groups are always present, often using the trance-like music of the *gamelan*. Emphasis is placed upon the ability of specific patterns of sound to heal—whether in the repeated *mantras* of meditation and yoga, or the repetitive music of the gamelan orchestra—especially in Ayurvedic healing traditions of Further India. Here, noting the instruments of later Islamic origin in combination with the music and sounds of ancient India, we can observe the transposition of these influences into the indigenous healing practices of Southeast Asia.

The gamelan orchestra generally consists of the following four types of drum and gong: *ketak*, *kenong*, *kempul*, and *gong*, arranged in a semicircle on the ground. The gong is used as a drum, by striking it with the palm of the hand. These are essentially Islamic instruments, the knobbed gong of Malaysia and Indonesia being distinct from the flat gong of China. The music is played in *kulingtang* rhythmic mode, rather than melodic mode. There are no scores and no conductors (and in this respect it is like a modern jazz jam session)—just a sense of circular, perpetual motion to carry the players along. The scale is *anahematonic* (five tones without semitones), and the polyphonic stratification is typical of all rice agriculture-based cultures. This music facilitates a trance-like state.

While in trance, the *bomoh* manifests a marked resting tremor, and may assume the spirits of the *Black Jin* (who represents the areas below the earth), the *Yellow Jin* (representing the mountains), and/or *Hanuman* (the white monkey of the *Ramayana*—*presbytis entellus*, a monkey of Southern Asia, has bristly white hairs on the crown and the face; the name "Hanuman" is derived from the Sanskrit *hanu*, "jaw," and *hanumat*, "having jaws"). The manifestation of these spirits themselves is drawn from the Sanskrit roots of Further India, and representations of the Buddha's healing realms (mountains, and under the earth), and they take the form of the *Jins* from Islam. Thus, in the healing trance, in real time, we can observe the successive influences of Further India, Greater China, and

Islam in images of health and healing, as if converging on an ancient archetype of celestial origins.

These *spirits* speak, sing and dance through the trance state with culturally significant gestures, similar to those observed in the Malay Opera and *Wayang Kulit* puppet theatre. The diagnosis is made by *divination*, which may or may not lead to exorcism. However, it is stressed that the sick individual is *not possessed* by a spirit but simply *made sick* by one. The spiritual ritual is to "weld the patient back together" after the illness has caused him or her to come apart.

Attempts are made today to draw these rituals into the currently predominant Islamic religion. *Fatima, the daughter of Mohammed the Prophet*, is said to have conducted the first spirit ritual therapy; the four companions of Mohammed played the four instruments. When completed, it is said, they threw the instruments into the sea, whence the Hebrews obtained them, going on to become the great healers of the ancient Islamic world.

The heritage of Adam and Eve, the original "peoples of the book," according to Islam, is also worked into the practice. In the Bible, the task of assigning names to the objects of nature is given to Adam and Eve, thereby allowing them to take place in this process of "creation." In the traditional formulation of disease causation, Satan gave birth only to the names of *Hontu* (superheated air) demons, which take on existence in the mind and go on to cause psychosomatic illness—the *spirit* component of disease. Also present is the Greco-Roman, Aristotelian concept of the four humors and the hot and cold qualities, ultimately incorporated into Arabic *Unani* medicine.

Despite these attempts to legitimize ethnomedical practices by making them congruent with Islam, Muslim officials do not recognize these healing rituals as part of health care. The situation is complicated by government ministries where some support the practice, others tolerate it, and still others oppose it. The attitude to traditional ethnomedical healing is very different in Vietnam, for example, as we shall see in Chapter 15.

The Islands of Indonesia

The Indonesian Archipelago consists of tens of thousands of islands ranging from the semi-continents of Java, Borneo (Kalimantan), and Sumatra, to "islands" within the islands, such as the Vedic Indian enclave of Bali. The indigenous populations and languages are similar to those of Malaya. Indonesia has the largest population of any Islamic country, numbering over 200 million, including millions of overseas Chinese and Indians, primarily in the urban areas.

Little is known of Indonesia earlier than 2000 years ago when, it appears, immigrants from Southeast Asia brought the secrets of bronze metallurgy, irrigation agriculture, and animal domestication, together with the cult of animism.

Chinese merchants and mariners visited the islands in search of precious gems. In the first century CE, the Han Chinese Emperor dispatched a delegation to Sumatra to obtain exotic zoological specimens, as recorded in Chinese texts. Written history in Indonesia itself began only in the fifth century with the early sequence of Hindu, Buddhist, and Islamic kingdoms, followed by the Portuguese, Spaniards, and finally, Dutch.

The persistent influences of Ayurveda and Islam

Islamic (Sufi) philosophy is a major influence in traditional medical practices in the Indonesian islands, of which the cultural center is Java. Indonesia was swept by the further reach of Islam in the fifteenth century, extending eastward to the island of Timor and northeastward to the southern Philippines. The earlier Vedic influences of Further India were swept back to the island of Bali, where they can be observed today.

In Java, traditional healing practice draws on a wide variety of symbols, roles, and interactional patterns which, as in Malay communal healing rituals, are not strictly medical. Concepts of personal identity, cosmology, power and knowledge are blended into a body of closely related theories explaining the origins of disease and motivating highly diverse treatment strategies. Medical pluralism is an inherent feature of Javanese traditional medicine. There are two primary modes of medical practice. One, practiced by holy men (Sufi *wali*), is based on Islamic mystical concepts of miracles and gnosis, clearly grafting the currently predominant Islamic religion onto healing practice. The other, practiced by *dukun* (curers), involves the use of sometimes (to Islamic authorities) morally suspect forms of magical power which has its own origins from celestial sources.

These two modes of medical practice can be seen to reflect a cosmological divide between light and dark, or, in the predominant religion's terms, between animism and Islam.

Chapter 14

The Philippine Islands

Archaeological and historical Chinese records document extensive and ongoing contacts with the Philippine Islands, largely through Chinese mariners and merchants. This contact increased after the Tang Dynasty (618–906 CE) when the overland Silk Road was impeded by incursions from the new Islamic wave emanating from Arabia, and China increasingly relied on trade by sea rather than overland. While trade expansion between Southeast Asia and China was due primarily to the spread of Chinese civilization for 1500 years, the arrival of Arab ships in China with goods from the Philippines began in 982 CE.

Contacts with China were intense during the Sung Dynasty (960–1280 CE) that followed. Contact also increased between the Philippines and mainland Southeast Asia, still primarily through the intermediary of Chinese maritime trade. During the Ming Dynasty (1368–1644) contacts with the northern islands of the Philippines (e.g. Luzon) remained strong, but the southern islands came directly under the influence of the expanding Islamic Empire from Indonesia. During the late Ming and Qing dynasties, trade contacts with China, and then the Americas, became dominated by the Spaniards with their famous "Manila galleons."

When the Spaniards first encountered the Malay peoples living in the Philippine Islands, they found a literate people who were versed in their own languages, with the ability to read and write.

The very first encounter with Ferdinand Magellan, a Portuguese mariner sailing for Spain, on his circumnavigation of the globe in 1521, was violent and ultimately fatal for Magellan at the hands of Chief Lapu-Lapu on the island of Cebu. Later Spanish clerics would document the more peaceful, literary aspects of life in the Philippines.

Nonetheless, not a single source of original Malay culture in the Philippines has remained. The materials used for writing on—rice paper, banana leaves, coco palm, and bamboo—were fragile and could not withstand the constant humidity, as well as periodic typhoons, frequent fires, and gnawing insects and rodents.

Spanish syncretism

Spanish clerics documented the practice of native healers they called *curanderos* (healers) and *herbolarios* (herbalists), but largely ignored the work of the mystic faith healers on the assumption that their *spiritual* work must somehow be associated with the devil. Therefore, the latter category of Philippine faith healing remained to be explored in the twentieth century, by which time the Filipinos themselves had melded traditional spiritual practices with the strong influence of the Roman Catholic Church (brought by the Spaniards) in a kind of unique, syncretic synthesis. Today many Filipino faith healers demonstrate syncretism with Roman Catholic religious concepts and figures.

Spiritual healing

The belief of the *Subanum*, an isolated tribe on the southern-most island of Mindanao (see page 153), is fairly typical. Illness was brought by *Pati-anak*, a demigod or devil which manifested as a beautiful child when held in the arms, but assumed the form of a worm when let loose and was to be avoided especially by pregnant women. The word *Pati-anak* is said to be derived from the Malay, *pati* meaning "dead," and *anak,* "child," although Blumentritt attributes a Sanskrit origin to the word *pati*, again showing the ancient influence of Further India in this part of the world. The imagery of the worm may derive from the Chinese *Ku* during the Zhou Dynasty, which was thought to embody the demons that were considered the causes of illness.

Among those groups which had more contact with outsiders over the course of history, this devil is called *Saitan, Sitan* (*Tagalogs*), or *Sidaan* (*Bisayas*), reflecting Islamic and Catholic etymology in the name of the devil.

All these influences appear to converge around the legend of the demon *kapre*, a cigar-smoking black giant (tobacco was introduced to the Philippines from the Americas by the Spanish in the 1500s). However, some folk healers are said to befriend the *kapre*, which may actually bring good fortune. Although usually silent, they have been said to warn of impending typhoons. The *kapre* is feared, but has affinity with the "friendly" Arabian genie from Islamic folklore. The Spanish were responsible for this demon's name, which is derived from the word *cafre* (an "infidel black African, or *Kaffir*"), through the Saracens who occupied Spain from about 700 to 1480 CE. According to legend, the *jinn* (*jinnee* or *genie*, plural) were created by Allah in a black, smokeless fire, thousands of years before Adam. They may show themselves as clouds or vast pillars, and can become visible in the shape of a man, jackal, wolf, lion, scorpion, or snake. In keeping with these ideas, the *kapre* is dispelled by reciting the *Paternoster* ("Our Father"), or naming the three members of the Holy Family, or running their names together, as in *Susmariosep* (Jesus, Mary, and Joseph) or even just *Mariosep*.

Another demon is the *mutya*, whose name is the Hindu word for "gem" or "jewel." It may convey strength, invisibility, or fertility.

Encounter with these demons may lead to *susto*, or the startle response, during which wind may enter the body, causing illness.

Skin deep

The Subanum tribe was also the subject of a classic medical ethnography by Charles O. Frake, based upon his fieldwork conducted in the 1950s. Frake found that members of the Subanum all agreed on the types of skin diseases that exist (which can be easily seen on the surface of the body), but that individuals disagreed on the diagnosis of the specific type of skin disease present in a given patient. This finding is a key observation of ethnomedicine: *types of disease that exist are generally known as part of the general knowledge of the culture,* but the *ability to correctly diagnose a specific disease in a given individual is highly dependent upon the skill of the individual who undertakes to treat the sick*—whether that skill is acquired by learning, apprenticeship, or divination. But there are healers in every society.

Healing ritual

Healing rituals in the Philippines bear similarities to those described for Malaya.

Here, a *katalonan* (healer/shaman) invokes divine power of celestial origin before conducing a *magdiwang* (healing ritual) for the sick. Offerings are shared in a communal meal, including pigs, chickens, fish, tortoise, oysters, rice, bananas, and aromatic spices. Often the most attractive girl was selected from among the participants to give a death blow to the sacrificial animal, perhaps like the Western myth of "beauty and the beast," and famously discussed in the pre-ethnomedical accounts of Sir James Frazer's *The Golden Bough.*

The healer enters a trance-like state and manifests resting tremors, as do the *bomoh* in Malaya. Instead of a gong, the healer holds a plate by the fingertips of the left hand, striking it with a string of seashells to make a bell-like sound.

Healing herbs

There were also medicine men (*herbolarios*) skilled in the use of medicinal plants. In 1669, the Spanish Jesuit missionary Francisco Ignacio Alcina first documented this indigenous pharmacopeia, followed in 1704 by the herbals of a Jesuit lay brother, George Joseph Camel, and in 1712 by Jesuit Father Pablo Clain. In a series of works written from 1751–1754, Jesuit Father Juan Delgado addressed the botany of these medicinal plants. In 1768 the Dominicans added their contribution with an herbal by Fernando de Santa Maria, which was used as late as 1923. The use of fly larvae (maggots) to treat infected wounds was among the effective knowledge of the *herbolario* that remained useful until this time.

The indigenous knowledge of the use of local herbs was considered appropriate and important by the Spanish, English (briefly), and later American rulers. The works of the Augustinian Father Ignacio de Mercardo in 1879, Tissot (*El aviso al pueblo*—"advice for the town," or essentially community public health, including the use of herbal medicines) in 1884, and Dr. Pardo de Tavera in 1892, were all published under Spanish royal patronage. With the arrival of the U.S. military in 1898, during and after the Spanish American War, these works were translated into English by Captain Jerome Thomas, Assistant Surgeon General, U.S.A.

Scientific studies on 17 selected medicinal plants were conducted by the first faculty of the University of the Philippines during the 1920s and 1930s. These remedies were found to be helpful for appendicitis, hydrophobia (the former name for rabies), chronic ulcers, acute laryngitis, and leprosy, and coconut and ylang-ylang oil were proved effective as a hair tonic—a fact which has not been lost on modern cosmetics manufacturers. A four-volume *Handbook on Philippine Medicinal Plants* is published by the University of the Philippines at Los Banos today.

Chapter 15

Mainland Vietnam, Thailand, and Burma

Vietnam is representative of the former French Indochina (which comprised Cambodia, Laos, and North and South Vietnam). For one thousand years, until 939 CE, Vietnam was politically part of the Chinese Empire, from the Han to the Sung dynasties. Except for language, Vietnam adopted virtually all of China's culture, including Confucianism, which had evolved during this era.

There continued a long period of mutual influence and respect with China, because Vietnam did indeed have Chinese culture and had been part of the "Middle Kingdom." When Vietnam was invaded by the Mongols of Kublai Khan in 1288, then ruling China under the Yuan Dynasty, and again in 1427, under the succeeding Ming Dynasty, Vietnam fought them back, but was careful to maintain political and cultural ties with China.

At the same time Vietnam looked beyond China to the north and expanded to the south, encountering the Khmer civilization. Throughout history, Vietnam remained largely an agrarian society, organized in villages where the communal good and the ethos of sharing were critical to maintaining health, as in Malaysia.

Despite the strong presence of Chinese medicine, in Vietnam being ill still means that one has offended a spirit, and a spiritual healer prescribes medicine and conducts ritual healing. The Vietnamese also believe in the law of *karma*, about which Buddhist teachings are invariably intermixed with those of Confucius. Good and evil influences can be projected and also can come home to roost, in terms of both illness and healing. "Projected vilification" is used to save face—for example, a woman scolding a dog in a village intends her words for a woman next door, who is inappropriately scolding and slapping her children. The only ones who do not know what is really happening are the naughty children and the poor dog.

Turning back to find a way forward

In the nineteenth century, the French introduced Roman Catholicism and Western medicine. During the twentieth century, developments in medicine were dominated by periods of armed conflict: with Japan (ending in 1945), with France (ending at Dien Bien Phu in 1954), and with the U.S., ending in 1975, since when North and South Vietnam have been united. During these extended periods of conflict, Vietnam was unable to obtain Western medicines.

Following Vietnam's war of independence from France, an official policy was first articulated by President Ho Chi Minh in 1954, asserting the importance of preserving and developing traditional medicine as a basic component of health care throughout the country, because a significant proportion of the population could not afford or obtain modern medicine.

A national heritage program in traditional medicine was established to ensure that the medical knowledge of experienced practitioners was gathered, recorded, and passed on to future generations through formal training programs. Simultaneously, a policy was developed to promote the modernization of traditional medicine and to incorporate it into health service provision, integrated with modern medicine. This policy was expanded and strengthened during the 1960s and 1970s, during the war between the North and the South. Emergency medical strategies were generated, including the development of a traditional medical program for the treatment of burns.

After several decades of pharmacognostic and toxicological research, the National Institute of Materia Medica in Hanoi developed a list of 1863 plants of known safety and efficacy in the treatment of common medical conditions. Traditional medicine now accounts for one third of all medical treatments provided (Institute of Materia Medica, Hanoi, 1990).

So, during the U.S.–Vietnam War for fully a decade from 1965 to 1975, North Vietnam actively redeveloped traditional ethnomedical resources to substitute for the Western medicines it could not obtain. After the unification of Vietnam under a Communist government and an extended period of political isolation from the West, the government continued to foster the use of traditional ethnomedicine. In light of the rich flora of Indochina, many medicinal plants provide effective (and cost-effective) remedies. In addition to the understanding that herbal remedies can be useful for the management of chronic medical conditions, as now accepted in the West, circumstances in Vietnam demonstrated the effectiveness of "alternative" remedies in emergency care, urgent care and acute care situations. In many ways the intentional and necessary *turning backward* of Vietnam toward ancient medical knowledge and resources may actually represent *a way forward* for developing countries, and for Western industrialized countries as well.

Appropriate medical technology

In Vietnamese peasant communities there is a common saying that traditional medicine costs one chicken, modern medicine costs one cow, and modern hospital treatment costs the whole herd (many cows). Rural people may have to travel for a day or more to reach a modern medical clinic or pharmacy. This results in lost wages, which is compounded by the cost of transport and the relatively high cost of medicines themselves.

At the basis of global concern about the ever-increasing cost of health care lies the issue of sustainability. Unlike Vietnam, many developing countries are mired in health care systems based on expensive, imported medicines and technologies, and continued reliance on these systems will result in health care costs consuming national finances and stifling national economic growth.

Industrialized countries are also struggling with decisions over who pays for health care—the state, employers, the public—and how the escalating costs of high-technology medicine can be controlled.

In the developing world, basic questions are now being asked about priorities in health expenditures and national economic development: how can countries address the health needs of their people without continuing to rely on expensive, imported pharmaceuticals? How can local, existing systems of health care be utilized to provide basic health services to rural and poor communities?

Increased attention is being paid to the potential of *locally available medicinal plants* and *inexpensive herbal medicines*, the key to diverse and distinct medical practices within the sphere of Greater China, in providing effective primary health care. This consideration has in turn raised concerns about the sustainable use of wild sources of medicinal plants, the conservation of biodiversity, appropriate forms of local cultivation and production, the safety and effectiveness of natural medicines, and the regulatory environment that should accompany the incorporation of traditional systems of health into national health care.

Thailand

Thailand's past remains a puzzle. There is a legend that the Thai originally came from China to get away from Kublai Khan during the Yuan Dynasty. The Khmer civilization of Angkor Wat was overtaken by the Thai in the 1430s, and the Lao kingdom by the Thai, Burmese, and Vietnamese. The original capital of Siam (Thailand) arose on the waters of the Chao Phraya River. In 1636 a Dutch trader described it as one of the largest cities south of China, "frequented by all Nations, and impregnable." But, after nearly half a millennium, it was sacked by the Burmese in 1767. The new center of Thai culture, Bangkok, was not founded until 1782.

Although Thailand (Siam) remained independent of Greater China, as well as subsequent British and French colonialism, massive immigration from China over the centuries has profoundly influenced Thai practices. The kings of Thailand's present Dynasty have Chinese ancestry. Although a relatively recent Dynasty in terms of Asian history, the Thai kings have combined the ancient Chinese traits of being considered divine, as well as compiling their histories retrospectively to cast great antiquity upon them. These attributes lend a divine and spiritual aspect to cultural traditions such as the practice of Thai medicine. In addition, the immigration of millions of Chinese has brought the systematic forms of Chinese medicine to widespread currency.

The spiritual and the practical exist side by side. A medical officer practicing on the Gulf of Siam saw his work endangered by Communist insurgents in the late 1960s. He appealed to King Bhumibol at the royal palace and spoke of roads, crops, psychology, the importance of the community, and spirits. The King gave the doctor funds but also commanded him, "I forbid you to become discouraged"—in the best tradition of the ancient Chinese Emperors.

Spirits inhabit everything in Thailand. In Bangkok, where a six-lane thoroughfare intersects with an eight-lane highway, stands a shrine to the Hindu deity Brahma, creator of the world, on the site of Erawan Hotel, name for the three-headed elephant ridden by another deity. There had been problems with construction of the new hotel, and Brahma is the patron of builders, since after all, he built the world. The Thai are in awe of spirits: spirits of places and things, spirits of living beings, from animals to the semi-divine (such as the King), and spirits of the dead and ancestors, mixing with Chinese as well as Hindu ideas.

In medicine the spiritual often overcomes the material. Village parents say they don't like to give medicines to their children that might offend them, because it is better not to hurt their feelings. Instead, babies only two weeks old are gently guided by their mothers to put their tiny palms together and raise them to their forehead in the traditional gesture of supplication. As the children grow older, they are taught elevation of the pressed palms to the different degrees: forehead for the Buddha and monks, the nose for superiors, and the chest for subordinates. Many ill children are treated by being taken to the lord abbot at the local wat, or Buddhist monastery. A fever is treated by the monk winding a thread around the child. Today, these Buddhist practices are as well established in Thailand as anywhere in the world.

Together with the spiritual emphasis, *materia medica* also has an important place in medical practice. A prized medicinal substance comes from birds' nests, the soup made from which, in the Chinese pharmacopeia, is said to lower blood pressure. Considerable organization and effort is required to harvest the nests from the vast limestone caverns that tunnel the Thai panhandle and islands, housing hordes of swifts, which secrete a glue-like substance in their mouths to mold delicate nests, sticking them fast to the most remote heights. Collectors harvest the first two nests of the birds, leaving the third for raising their young.

Thai medical concepts

Traditional Thai medicine (TTM), as it is practiced today, lies at the intersection of many disparate medical traditions, from Indian Ayurvedic and yogic traditions to traditional Chinese medical influences. It draws on each for inspiration, in the process carving out its own unique niche in the medical world. Some observers have tried to separate the tradition into formal "medical" and informal "folk healing" practices, or to unify all of the distinct beliefs under a single theoretical umbrella. However, in actuality Thai medicine is an amalgam of both formal practices documented in writing and given credence by the royal court and the Thai government, and informal "folk" practices handed down orally and practiced outside of the government sphere. Its diversity and knowledge cannot easily be pigeon-holed or grouped within Ayurvedic medicine or TCM.

The Thai notion is that of holistic being based on the idea that human life is composed of three essences—body, mind/

heart (*citta*), and energy—which constantly flow into each other and create the "circle of life." The body represents the physical self, the *citta* encompasses the complete inner self—thoughts, emotions, and the spirit—and energy is the glue that binds the two selves, somewhat analogous to the Chinese notion of *qi*. This energy is an intangible force which flows throughout the body along 72,000 different channels (*sen*) (Salguero 2003). According to traditional Thai medicine, disease arises from an imbalance in these three interconnected essences. In this way disease is not merely a physical phenomenon, but also an emotional, psychological and spiritual event. All diseases affect all three essences, and so all TTM treatment must address all three in order to maintain a proper balance (Salguero 2006). These three essences give rise to the three branches of Thai medicine, the goal of which is maintaining a physical, emotional, spiritual, and mental equilibrium (Figure 15.1).

Body
Physical structures: cells, molecules, atoms

Physiological processes: hormones, metabolism, aging

Energy
Relatively physical manifestations: electricity, magnetism, heat

Relatively mental/spiritual manifestations: mood, general energy level

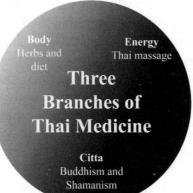

Citta (Mind–Heart)
Mind: intellect, beliefs, thoughts, reason, learning

Heart: emotion, intuition, faith, spirituality

Figure 15.1 The three branches of Thai medicine and the "circle of life"

Traditional Thai medicine resembles other Asian traditional medical practices in its holistic view of health and focus on the relations among the physical, spiritual and emotional selves. It parallels Chinese medicine, where energy balance is accomplished through *qi gong*, *t'ai chi* or acupuncture; *citta* balance is maintained through Mahayana Buddhist and Taoist practices. It also resembles Indian Ayurvedic medicine, where energy balance is maintained through yoga; *citta* balance is maintained through Hindu practices. In traditional Thai medicine, body balance is maintained through herbal remedies and a proper diet, *citta* balance is maintained through the practice of Buddhism and Thai animism, and energy balance is maintained through Thai massage.

The exact ways in which each of these essences interacts and affects well-being is of little consequence to the TTM practitioner. He does not search for scientific substantiation of his beliefs, or seek to understand the rationale behind the various therapies, but takes them as a given. He works instead to help patients maintain existing balance, or restore balance when it is disrupted, by prescribing herbal remedies, administering herbal ointments, offering manipulative massage therapies, or reciting various chants or incantations. Balance can be upset by a variety of different factors, ranging from environmental or climate factors to dietary factors, from emotional factors to interpersonal relationship factors, from genetic factors to other physical factors. Different TTM practitioners, both formal and informal, are trained to address different aspects of the imbalance by means of different therapies.

To become a full-fledged TTM doctor, as recognized by the royal court and the government, requires three years of official training in herbalism and traditional diagnostics. Massage therapy can be taken during a fourth, optional year. In 2005 there were over 37,000 formally recognized TTM practitioners in Thailand and over 80 percent of hospitals incorporated some form of TTM into their practice (Chokevivat *et al.* 2005; Chokevivat and Chuthaputti 2005). In addition to formal TTM practitioners, there is also a host of different "folk" healers who operate outside of the formal realm to treat both natural and supernatural causes of disease using various ceremonies, charms, amulets, tattoos, and holy incantations (Brun 2003; Chuakul *et al.* 1997). These formal and informal practitioners compose the pluralistic medical landscape of Thailand—allowing patients choices from among allopathic, traditional or folk healers who best suit their spiritual, psychological, and physical needs.

Thai herbalism: treating the body

The principal goal of Thai medicine is balancing, not only amongst the different essences, but also amongst the different elements that compose the physical body. According to Thai medicine, the physical body comprises the same four elements that make up the universe—Earth, Fire, Water, and Air—and the goal of herbalism is to ensure that these elements are kept in proper proportion to each other—that they are balanced. This concept is similar to the Ayurvedic notions of cosmology and the body constitutions. The organs of the body can be ascribed to different elemental categories, based on their qualities and properties (Table 15.1). Disease develops when any of these elements is in excess, depleted, or absent (Table 15.2).

Table 15.1 The four body elements, their qualities, and the organs they affect

Element	Quality	Organs
Earth	Solid	Skin, muscles, tendons, bones, viscera, fat, other solid organs
Water	Liquid	Blood, eyes, phlegm, saliva
Air	Movement	Respiration, digestion, excretion, motion of limbs and joints, sexuality, aging
Fire	Heat	Body temperature, circulatory system, metabolism

Table 15.2 Effects of excess, depletion, or absence of the four elements within the physical body

Element (sample organ)	Excess	Depletion	Absence
Earth (muscle)	Cramps, stress	Weakness, convulsions, poor elasticity in muscles	Inflammation, pain, bruising, spasms, fatigue, muscular atrophy, paralysis
Water (saliva)	Excess saliva in mouth	Thick saliva, difficulty in chewing and swallowing	Dry, painful, bloody mouth, bad breath, dry throat, extreme thirst
Wind (circulation)	High blood pressure, headache	Low blood pressure, fatigue, faintness	Circulatory failure, unconsciousness, paralysis
Fire (metabolism)	Fast deterioration of cells and organs	Thick skin and tongue	Bleeding and circulatory problems; blood vessel constriction, brain atrophy, heart failure, death

These four elements provide the essential link between patient symptoms and herbal treatments. A patient's symptoms correspond to an excess or depletion of any of these elements, so once the element concerned is identified, the body systems involved can be treated by means of herbal remedies prescribed accordingly. In TTM practice, analogous to some Ayurvedic and Siddha practices in India, as well as Chinese food/flavor guidelines, pharmacological substances are classified by ten categories of flavor or taste—astringent (*fat*), oily (*man*), salty (*khem*), sweet (*wan*), bitter (*khom*), toxic (*mao-buea*), sour (*priao*), hot (*phet*), aromatic (*hom yen*), and bland. Each taste quality has a different effect (either increasing or decreasing) on each of the elements, and hence a different effect on body functioning. Since herbs each have a distinctive taste, different herbal remedies can be used to treat different elemental imbalances (Table 15.3 and Table 15.4).

Symptoms often manifest simultaneously as combined excess and depletion of different elements, which need to be teased apart in order for the proper treatments to be administered. As a result, this process of elemental diagnosis is more of an art than a science—one reason why several years of training are required to become a certified TTM practitioner.

Table 15.3 Tastes and their effects on the elements

Taste	*Increases*	*Decreases*
Astringent	Air	Earth, Water, Fire
Oily (nutty)	Earth, Water, Fire	Air
Salty	Earth, Water, Fire	Air
Sweet	Earth, Water	Air, Fire
Bitter	Air	Earth, Water, Fire
Toxic (nauseating)	Air, Fire	Earth, Water
Sour	Water, Fire	Earth, Air
Hot (spicy)	Air, Fire	Earth, Water
Bland	Earth, Water, Air	Fire
Aromatic (cool)	Earth, Water, Air	Fire

As in China, Thai herbalism practice rarely uses single herbs as a treatment. Rather they are prescribed as compounds consisting of multiple ingredients, classified as (1) the *main* ingredients, (2) *auxiliary* herbs which support the action of the main ingredients, (3) *controlling* herbs which are used to reduce toxicity and control the compound and coloring, and (4) *flavoring* herbs which are used to make the concoction more palatable. Herbs can be made into fluid extracts, infusions, alcoholic macerates, pills, or tablets, or delivered through an herbal sauna bath, with each herb having a different ideal preparation.

Table 15.4 The ten tastes and their therapeutic uses

Taste	Action	For treatment of…	Contraindications
Astringent	Hemostatic, topical astringent, topical antiseptic, diuretic, hepatic, digestive, stomachic, antirheumatic	Internal bleeding wounds, dysentery and other diarrhea, pus, discharge, water retention, liver and stomach disease, sluggish digestion, arthritis	Constipation
Oily	Nutritive tonic	Impaired strength, energy, vitality, chronically low body temperature, stiff and sore joints, muscles and tendons, skin disease, itching	Obesity
Salty	Laxative, antiseptic	Constipation, flatulence, sluggish digestion, excessive mucous in digestive tract, mouth sores	Chronic thirst, dehydration
Sweet	Nutritive tonic, demulcent	Impaired strength, energy and vitality, chronic disease, low immunity, chronic fatigue and exhaustion, convalescence from disease or injury, asthma, sore throat, cough	Diabetes, hypoglycemia, gum disease, tooth decay
Bitter	Bitter tonic, tonic for blood and bile, antipyretic, cholagogue, hepatic, lymphatic	Disease of blood and bile, parasites and infection in blood, fever, dengue, malaria, low immune system functioning	Chronic fatigue

	Actions	Indications	Cautions
Toxic	Detoxifier, antihelminthic, vermifuge, purgative, analgesic, antiseptic	Systemic infections, tetanus, venereal diseases, cholera, dysentery, diarrhea, gastro-intestinal parasites, infections, festering wounds	These herbs have a nauseating taste/smell and should only be used with caution
Sour	Expectorant, pectoral, refrigerant, nervine, diuretic	Congested mucous, respiratory infections, asthma, bronchitis, cough, fever, infection of blood, lymph, sluggish circulation, clarity of mind and senses	
Hot	General stimulant, digestive, carminative, cardiac, expectorant, aphrodisiac, anti-inflammatory, antispasmodic, diaphoretic	Low immunity, chronic fatigue, sluggish digestion, indigestion, flatulence, constipation, sinusitis, common cold, nasal congestion, sore or cramping muscles	Fever, hypertension, cardiac disease
Aromatic	Cardiac tonic, hepatic, pectoral, nervine, sedative, calmative, stimulant, female tonic, detoxifier, diuretic	Heart disease, circulatory problems, disease of liver and lungs, chronic anxiety, tension or stress, hypertension, psychological and emotional imbalances, chronic fatigue, exhaustion, depression, mental clarity and well-being, post-partum depression	Aromatics are typically administered through sauna or steam, which should be avoided by those suffering from fever, heart disease or high blood pressure
Bland		Food or chemical poisoning, chronic thirst	

While there are a handful of different herbs unique to Thailand and the practice of TTM, the vast majority—almost 80 percent—of herbs found in TTM texts are also found in the classic Ayurvedic pharmacopoeia; most of the remaining 20 percent come from popular Chinese remedies. In this way, Thai herbalism draws on multiple external influences, combining them in a multitude of different recipes, which make them uniquely Thai. Thai herbalism builds on existing Asian medical traditions, but adds to them and the ways in which they can be used to diagnose and treat the physical body. The vast majority of Thai herbal recipes have been transmitted orally from one generation to the next. As in China and Vietnam, the government of Thailand has launched a massive effort to recover this evanescent Thai knowledge and record it before it is lost forever.

Thai massage: treating the energy

Thai herbalism provides a way of balancing the elements of the physical body; Thai massage provides a way to maintain the flow of vital energy throughout that body and to ensure the continual connection between the physical and spiritual selves. Thai massage (*nuat boran*) is a unique blend of both Indian tantric yoga and Chinese acupressure and involves the therapist both manipulating the patient's body into various yogic positions and stimulating specific pressure points along the bodies *"sen"* or vessels.

Although Thai herbalism practice has been standardized across the country, Thai massage differs drastically from one region to the next, from one school to the next. Each school teaches different *sen* lines and different massage techniques. Moreover, Thai massage is often practiced by informally trained healers who have learned the art orally, without the theory behind it.

Thai massage can be used both as a preventative measure, to strengthen a patient's immunity, increase circulation and lymphatic functioning and ensure adequate energy flow, and as a form of treatment, by stimulating and relaxing a patient's mind and body to promote the natural healing process and to free up trapped energy which may be preventing proper bodily functioning. It can also be used as an *adjunct* therapy to promote healing alongside herbal remedies or other allopathic treatments. Because massage is an art of working with energy, rather than with the body *per se*, traditional massage practitioners are not guided by anatomical structures, but instead follow the patient's energy meridians, guided by intangible forces.

Thai massage is governed by a Buddhist code of ethics which all practitioners must follow, both inside and outside of their practice. One of the most important aspects of the healing process is the compassionate *intent* of the healer, who must have a deep awareness of himself and his client in order to adequately perform the practice. This compassionate state of mind is referred to as *metta*, which translates directly into "loving kindness." *Metta*, in conjunction with proper techniques, guides the healer in his massage performance. In order to conjure up *metta*, every practitioner begins his session with a prayer to Shivago Komarpaj, who was Buddha's doctor and is said to be the founder of traditional Thai medicine:

> We invite the spirit of our founder,
> the Father Doctor Shivago, who taught us through his saintly life.
> Please bring to us knowledge of nature,
> and show us the true medicine in the universe.
> Through this prayer, we request your help,
> that through our hands
> you will bring wholeness and health to the body of our client.
> The god of healing dwells in the heavens high, while mankind remains in the world below.
> In the name of the founder,
> may the heavens be reflected in the earth,
> so that this healing medicine may encircle the world.
> We pray for the one whom we touch,
> that we will be happy and that any illness will be released from him.

Combining formal and folk practices

Thai herbalism and Thai massage only scratch the surface of the formal practice of TTM, which is documented in books and on stone tablets such as those found at Wat Pho in Bangkok. These formalized practices and the theories behind them draw very heavily on influences from India, China, and other surrounding nations. In fact, in many respects these theories and traditions evolved in the way they did—to resemble Ayurvedic, yogic, and Chinese practices—because of pressure by the Thai government to standardize and legitimize them in the way these other medical practices have now been legitimized. Grounding TTM in theory and documenting it in books gained for it a credence it had once lacked, and so it became a formal healing art. However, in the process of standardizing and formalizing TTM, a lot of important traditional "folk" practices were left out of the literature and out of the training. These "folk" practices have both shaped traditional Thai medicine and given it a unique flair—and set Thai medicine apart from Chinese medicine and Ayurveda.

On the one hand, formal TTM emphasizes the internal world and the internal balance amongst the different essences and elements that comprise the physical body. In this light, disease is seen as an internal imbalance. On the other hand, TTM also deals, in a less formal sense, with the external world and external spiritual forces which can cause disease or malady. This aspect of Thai medicine, dealing with the cosmos, like the ancient shamanic traditions, is not the purview of formally trained TTM doctors, but rather the realm of "folk" healers who use magical powers or spiritual allies to treat or protect patients. Together these two brands of Thai medicine can address both the internal and external, natural and supernatural causes of disease. According to Thai beliefs, it is even possible for these external forces to upset internal balance, so it is important to understand not only the formal practices of Thai herbalism and Thai massage, but also the informal practices of the *mo tjalo* (folk practitioners), *mo du* (fortune tellers), *mo song* (diviners), *mo phi* (spirit mediums), and *mo wicha* (controllers of magical powers).

While folk healing traditions are not based on learned ideas or coherent theories, beliefs about the supernatural realm are deeply embedded in the fabric of Thai culture and play an important part in Thai medicine. Spirit mediums can be used to maintain harmony between the human and spirit worlds, to ensure that the needs of spirits are met so that they do not harm human beings. Other spirit mediums are said to have the ability to pacify ghosts or demons, using consecrated water and holy chants to drive them from the bodies of possessed individuals. Still other folk healers are said to be able to call back a soul which has been dislodged or lost, and in doing so, restore health to that individual. *Tham khwan*, or "calling of the soul," usually involves offerings, chanting and the binding of the patient's right wrist with consecrated thread to tie the soul metaphorically to the body, once it has returned.

It is not just folk healers, however, who use incantations or call on spirits to influence health. Even traditionally trained Thai herbalists recite sacred chants over their medicinal concoctions to give them additional spiritual potency, and massage therapists call on the spirits of past teachers to guide them in their treatment work.

Thai medicine, then, is an amalgam of both formal practices which require formal training and follow requisite courses, and informal, folk practices, which are practiced by village "folk" healers and transmitted orally. In making decisions about treatment a patient rarely sees the therapeutic options available as mutually exclusive. It is often the case that people seek a combination of different allopathic, folk and formal TTM treatments in addressing their maladies—further blurring the lines that separate one practice from the next. So, rather than lumping all TTM practices under a single unified theory, it helps to understand under what circumstances each practice is most suitable because, more often than not, dealing with ailments requires treatment of both natural and supernatural causes of illness—by restoring balance amongst all essences and elements using herbs, acupressure, chants, and allopathic medicines in succession.

In this way, Thai medicine embodies the merger of medical concepts and practices from Greater China with Further India, as well as relying on local resources.

On the Burmese–Thai border

Although historically China did not ultimately incorporate Burma, Cambodia, Laos, and Thailand into its Empire, as it had Vietnam, the influences of the Middle Kingdom were strong in practical matters such as weights and measures, and medicine. Literature and art show the influences of Further India and the teachings of the Buddha, equally claimed by China and East Asia as well. For example, the traditional national Burmese dress, the *longyi*, consists of a wrap-around skirt from India and a short formal jacket with three pockets and cloth buttons from China. Tribute to the Emperor of China was paid by the Burmese through most of history.

In contrast to present-day Thailand, not much is known today about the state of traditional medical practices in Burma, thanks to the isolationist and repressive regime in power there since 1962—what some have called a *"ne win"* situation— aside from anthropological ethnographies from the 1930s and 1950s, by Edmund Leach and others. A recent example among Burmese refugees on the Thai border (notable for the bridge on the River Kwai, made famous by David Lean's film) illustrates two principles that have been presented throughout this book: the importance of the local *materia medica*, and the ability to adapt and incorporate new resources into medical practice.

Forced migration due to war or persecution of political dissidents can remove people from mainstream medical care and create increased reliance on medical practices from their own cultural traditions, even in the face of unfamiliar local *materia medica*. In one study of Burmese refugees at the Thai–Burmese border, extensive use of traditional medicine was found, despite official views that there was little or no traditional medicine use among these displaced groups.

Bureaucratic Western aid agencies set the global agenda for refugees, and ultimately determine the fate of refugees' health and well-being. By not looking at traditional systems of health care, these agencies are overlooking a valuable sustainable resource, as well as contributing to the loss of important cultural knowledge. By contrast, through harnessing this knowledge and its practices, refugee health agencies could help facilitate new global strategies for coping, and new prospects for development.

As we shall see in Part IV, Chinese medicine today represents a global system of medicine that is forging the integration between traditional healing and modern health care.

PART IV

❧

Chinese Medicine in the West and Worldwide

Chapter 16

Chinese Medicine in the Twentieth and Twenty-First Centuries

In China, during the twentieth century, medical practice was redefined. With the formation of the Republic of China in 1911, reformers attempted to institute sweeping cultural changes, pushing aside remnants of the old empire to make way for the modern age. In medicine, that meant trying to replace traditional practices with new ones based on contemporary science.

The Imperial Medical College was closed, and from 1914 to 1936, both Chinese nationalists (under *Sun Yat Sen* and *Chiang Kai Shek*) and Marxists (under *Mao Tse Tung*, or *Zedong*) sought to "reform" practitioners of traditional medicine. Even the name came under attack: what had always been called simply "medicine" (*yi*), was now called "Chinese medicine" (*zhong yi*), and those practices deemed "unscientific" according to new twentieth-century medicine were rejected. *Zhong yi* redefined traditional Chinese medicine as the form in which it is practiced today.

The aspects of traditional medicine that survived as *zhong yi* were later appropriated by Chinese Communists in an effort to build a strong, low-cost medical infrastructure for the new nation's vast underserved population.

In 1958 Chairman Mao declared, "Chinese medicine is a great treasure house! We must uncover it and raise its standards!" The system of traditional medicine was to be rehabilitated by Communist modernists who would appropriately "discover" a primitive dialectical ("Marxist") logic within its theoretical underpinnings. *The Revised Outline of Chinese Medicine* stated that "Yin–yang and the Five Phases are ancient Chinese philosophical ideas. They are spontaneous, naive materialist theories that also contain elementary dialectical ideas."

Today, *zhong yi* exists in China as a parallel medical system, integrating biomedical elements while retaining fidelity to the traditional concepts of Chinese medicine; both inpatient and outpatient medical care is delivered from large, well-equipped hospitals, as well as from private clinics and pharmacies. Educational programs emphasize *acupuncture* and *herbal medicine*, and range from an undergraduate technical certificate to PhD programs. Most independent practitioners enter the field with a five-year medical baccalaureate degree (MB/BS) that is gained following high school.

Today TCM is a global entity that is quite distinct from its premodern counterpart. The chief modalities that have come to characterize TCM include acupuncture, moxibustion, herbal medicine, dietary therapy, *tui na* (massage), and *qi gong*. Concepts of *qi*, its cultivation, and flow are critical to each of these modalities. Moreover, the meridians or channels through which *qi* flows, or in which it can be blocked, or become stagnant, are key sites in considerations of pathology and therapeutic intervention.

While concepts of *qi* in TCM theory and practice seem similar to those of classical or premodern forms of Chinese medicine, there has been a transition in the definition and uses of *qi* in contemporary TCM texts. In the *Suwen*, for instance, *qi* was defined as a cosmic force, as well as a bodily substance. The concept of *qi* in post-1949 medical texts, however, tends to reflect solely physiological dimensions and to emphasize *qi* primarily as a bodily substance like blood and other bodily fluids. This change is due in part to the medicalization of practice and the discourses of scientific Marxism, where social, environmental, and phenomenological meanings of the body and its forms are reconfigured into more material categories with physical properties, such that the body is seen less as an energetic entity and is redefined in a form that is more predictable and, presumably, controllable.

Qi gong in the twenty-first century

Nowadays elements of social control are evident in developments involving the practice of *qi gong*. During the late twentieth century *qi gong*, or the practice of breathwork and healing through cultivating one's *qi*, became an immensely popular form of exercise and healing in crowded, urban areas, especially in China itself. Throughout major cities and towns one could always find practitioners in the early dawn in parks, on sidewalks, near public buildings, on campuses, and even in streets, participating in daily regimens of *qi gong* exercise. Broad social awareness of this practice was reflected in mainstream state newspapers as well as popular novels. *Qi gong* was understood as fostering the movement of *qi* through the body, either by internal visualization and meditation, or through external bodily practices involving physical movement. Seen as more than a merely physical substance, *qi* was embraced as cosmological energy by practitioners and masters. Such popular views of *qi* as a healing force seemed to return to earlier, more "traditional" ideas of *qi*, according to which individuals could draw upon or embody its transformative powers as present in the environment and cosmos, rather than merely in a body confined by everyday spaces. Most *qi gong* manuals tend to echo traditional medical texts in discussion of *yin–yang* and how *qi* is manifest with these dual qualities.

Experiencing *qi* was a central component of practice that all *qi gong* practitioners encountered and discussed on a daily basis. However, since there are multiple forms of *qi*, the ways in which *qi* was invoked to describe practice varied widely.

Despite the variety of styles and practice, *qi gong* can be distinguished into two types—*external* and *internal*. The external form, based on *waidan* (外丹) cultivation principles, tends to emphasize "hard" *qi* and "hard" bodies that can withstand much force and perform superhuman powers. This *martial arts* form tends to be practiced not so much in public parks as in arenas, or military compounds, or by acrobatic troupes (and more by men).

The internal and meditative form, based on *neidan* (內丹) cultivation, was pursued by practitioners of all backgrounds (particularly women) as such forms helped to promote the circulation and transformation of *qi* as crucial steps toward enhancing vitality.

In the 1980s, the initial post-Mao period prior to the formation of a massive market economy and global pharmaceutical industry (which came later, in the 1990s), *qi gong* emerged simultaneously as both a private act for individuals and a public performance for masters. In contrast to previous decades where socialized medicine attended to the masses with a focus on public health, the emergence of *qi gong* in the 1980s was linked to the desire for self-care and individualized forms of healing and daily practice. Elderly people could address their complaints of rheumatism or arthritis, sufferers of neurasthenia or chronic pain could seek relief, and parents of children with congenital disorders could seek help when no other options could be found in either traditional Chinese medicine or biomedicine. *Qi gong* became a practice that promised release and hope; and, whether in parks or in stadiums, it became acceptable to cry openly or express fervent belief in something that was not state ideology. As some forms of *qi gong* began to overlap with *Daoist*, *Buddhist*, and other spiritual practices, references to *qi gong* as a religion or *New Age spiritualism* also appeared.

During the 1990s official state debates about *qi gong* situated it clearly apart from popular *qi gong*. While testimonial accounts of *qi gong* healing continued, there were calls to differentiate between "real" (*zheng*) and "false" (*jia*) *qi gong*. There was an attempt to distinguish those individuals who claimed to be masters, and healed for lucrative purposes, from those with "true" abilities, practicing "more orthodox and uniform" forms. A state-appointed bureau to regulate *qi gong* used scientific discourse about *qi gong* (*kexue de qi gong*) as a means to cleanse and discipline the ranks of "false" masters.

Taken out of context, *qi gong* could be considered essentially apolitical in nature, but, as in the West, the Chinese social-political body has at times unconsciously expressed what is not culturally or politically acceptable. This manifestation has arguably been the case with *qi gong*. (The word itself, as having a standardized meaning, was actually *created* by government in 1953.) With the lifting of many restrictions in China in the 1990s, more elaborate, spontaneous forms of *qi gong* enabled expression of much that had remained repressed under Mao (in a culture that is in any event not overly given to emotional self-expression).

In the words of one commentator, *qi gong* practice became "a symptom of repressed desires" (*xu*), and with the rise of the *falun gong* (法輪功) protest movement, *qi gong* was very definitely politicized (as previously during the movement leading to the Boxer uprising of 1900). The body politic has influenced the understanding of the effects of medical practices on the human body, from ancient times to the present. Medical practices, east and west, reflect the cultural, economic, political, and social contexts in which they arise. This ancient and rich mixture in China has given rise to a much fuller and comprehensive practice of *qi* manipulation (including acupuncture) than what has generally been accounted for, or rendered, in Western interpretations.

Chapter 17

Chinese Medicine
in Europe and
North America

East meets West

During these rises and falls of traditional medical practice in China itself, the sphere of Greater Chinese influence extended even into Europe and North America. As Marco Polo brought back aspects of Chinese technology to Europe in the Middle Ages, later developments introduced specific medical practices.

The medical use of acupuncture in Europe dates from the middle of the seventeenth century. The work of Willem Ten Rhyne (1647–1690) in this area culminated in the publication in 1683 of *Dissertatio de Arthritide*: *Mantissa Schematica*: *de Acupunctura*: *et Orationes Tres*, based on information gathered during his service in Japan as a physician for the *Dutch East India Company*. The *German* physician Kämpfer, who also traveled with the Dutch East India Company and spent time in *Japan*, contributed his observations.

In *France* the Jesuit Du Halde published a text that included a detailed discussion of Chinese medicine in 1735 (Hsu 1989). Later, in 1939, the publication of Soulié de Morant's

L'acupuncture Chinoise provided extensive discussion of the practice of acupuncture based on direct translation, observation, and actual practice by the author. This text was rooted in de Morant's exposure to the medicine of China in that country from 1901 to 1917.

England saw the publication of J. M. Churchill's *A Description of Surgical Operations Peculiar to Japanese and Chinese* in 1825. Among early notable English acupuncturists are Drs Felix Mann and Sidney Rose-Neil, both of whom began their explorations of acupuncture in the late 1950s, and who have influenced its development substantially in English-speaking countries. J. R. Worsley, a physical therapist, who began his studies of acupuncture in 1962, came to have a substantial impact on the perceptions of many practitioners in England and the United States. He visited Hong Kong and Taiwan for a brief period and then became a part of the study group established by Rose-Neil. Worsley went on to create the College of Traditional Chinese Acupuncture and two schools in the *United States*.

In 1826, Benjamin Franklin Bache (great-grandson of Benjamin Franklin) had become one of the first American physicians to use acupuncture in his practice. Ten Rhyne's text was a part of Sir William Osler's library, and in his *Principles and Practice of Medicine* Osler prescribes acupuncture for lumbago. Osler practiced, and his influence was felt, in Canada, the U.S., and Great Britain.

Apart from occasional explorations by the conventional medical community, the traditional medicine of China has been practiced in the United States since the middle of the nineteenth century. Herbal merchants, entrepreneurs, and physicians accompanied Chinese who sold their labor in the United States. The practice of "the China Doctor" *Doc Ing Hay*, in the town of John Day, Oregon, is probably one of the most famous. *Ah Fong Chuck*, who came to the United States in 1866, became the first licensed practitioner of that medicine in the United States in 1901, when he successfully won a medical license through legal action in Idaho.

With the strengthening of medical practice acts, the interruption of the herb supply from China, and the advent of World War II, these practices disappeared or retreated into

Chinatowns. Although the exposure of millions of Americans, Australians, Canadians, and Europeans to Greater China during and after World War II, the Korean War, and the Vietnam War, led to profound influences on popular philosophy (culminating in vast cultural movements in the West in the 1960s), they did not directly lead to expansion of Chinese medical practices. Then the leader of the "free world," Richard Nixon, went to China in 1971.

Coming back into practice

With President Nixon's "re-opening" of China in 1971, substantial attention became focused on acupuncture, the traditional medicine of China, and its regional variants, as a result of *New York Times* journalist James Reston's highly publicized appendectomy and postoperative care during this diplomatic mission (see the box on the following page). This event turned a spotlight on varieties of medical practice that had been largely confined to Asia and the Chinatowns of the West. Increased visibility led to substantial public interest in acupuncture, and gradually to the licensure and development of training programs in the West. Today in the U.S., for example, almost all states (including the District of Columbia) license, certify, or register the practice of acupuncture and a range of other activities, including herbal medicine, by non-physicians. There are over 60 programs in the United States offering training in acupuncture and Oriental medicine.

In the modern West, there has been clear interest in the available range of expressions of the medical tradition of China: *European* interpretations of the application of *Five Phase Theory, Korean* constitutional acupuncture, traditional Chinese medicine (acupuncture, herbs, *qi gong*, and *tui na*), *Japanese meridian* therapy, and special family lineages within the Chinese tradition are all taught and practiced. This willingness to accept and explore the traditional and contemporary interpretations of traditional Chinese medicine has led to the emergence of the concept of "oriental medicine" as an umbrella term for the global domain of practice in this area.

Nixon in China

"For anesthesia, she has been given a mild sedative and a small amount of narcotic…and acupuncture needles… The young woman is awake, but doesn't flinch under the surgeon's knife… 'How are you doing?' I ask through an interpreter. 'Okay.'"

Acupuncture and traditional Chinese Medicine, described here by journalist Bill Moyers in his book and TV series *Healing and the Mind*, are probably the best known but least understood of the complementary and alternative therapies used in Europe and North America. Acupuncture had returned to the attention of the English-speaking public in 1971, when *New York Times* journalist James Reston, visiting China as part of President Nixon's press corps, required an emergency appendectomy. Reston suffered postoperative complications including abdominal pain and was successfully treated with acupuncture and moxibustion. Reston found his experience so remarkable that he wrote a column on it for the *New York Times*, introducing millions of new readers in the West to this uniquely Asian approach to treatment. Today, acupuncture is a household word in the West, yet few truly understand what it means, because acupuncture and other forms of traditional Chinese Medicine are based on the profoundly different conceptions of health, the body, even the nature of life itself.

The extent to which Chinese medicine has come to be viewed as an established therapeutic practice in the West was illustrated by a regulatory action recently taken by the United States Food and Drug Administration (FDA). After a series of reports of adverse events surrounding the use of dietary supplements containing ephedra (or originally, the Chinese *ma huang*; see pages 62–64) in weight loss regimes and athletic training (neither of which can, in any sense, be considered to constitute the practice of

Chinese medicine), the U.S. FDA considered itself compelled to act. On 6 February 2004 the FDA issued a final rule prohibiting the sale of dietary supplements containing ephedrine alkaloids (ephedra) "because such supplements present an unreasonable risk of illness or injury." Curiously enough, it was specifically stated that the "scope of the rule does not pertain to traditional Chinese herbal remedies." While the logistics of honoring this exemption have yet to be worked out, it signifies a definite acknowledgement of the professional practice of Chinese herbal medicine today.

Worldwide dissemination and integration

Today, China's traditional medicine is practiced, in various forms, all over the world. Sometimes it follows the contemporary patterns of traditional Chinese medicine; elsewhere its practice is deeply influenced by local custom, preference, or regional variation, as in Southeast Asia. Through vast communities of overseas Chinese throughout Southeast Asia (see Chapters 11, 12, and 13), it is also available alongside the indigenous healing traditions of the hinterlands.

Traditional Chinese medicine is practiced in a range of clinical settings. In China, large hospitals entirely devoted to its practice offer acupuncture, herbal medicine, and *tui na*, on both an inpatient and outpatient basis. It is not unusual to see a large outpatient facility treating 20 patients simultaneously in the same space. Smaller practices and even roadside stands are also common. Herbal prescriptions can be obtained from a Chinese herb store in almost any country that has a significant Chinese population. In *Japan*, small hospitals, large clinics, and private offices are typical settings.

In the *West* the demands of record-keeping, insurance billing, biomedical screening processes, and office hygiene often produce a setting that looks very much like a typical physician's office—except for the presence of such unusual features as acupuncture needles, moxa fluff, and herbs. Medical practice that meets cultural expectations is generally most desired by clients. In the U.S., a licensed physician can become a licensed acupuncturist in most states by completing a six-week training course in acupuncture. Although such physicians know little about Chinese medical cosmology, vital energy or "celestial healing," research shows that their "formulary" version of acupuncture is nonetheless effective.

Acupuncture delivered in a sterile environment by physicians in white coats works for many Westerners. In contrast, a Chinese person living in the West will not seek care from a "six-week" Western doctor but from a "sixth-generation" practitioner in Chinatown, knowing that many of the most effective secrets of successful acupuncture treatment are passed down through generations of acupuncturists.

As in Chinatowns worldwide, Chinese medicine is available in pluralistic health care environments, existing as a choice among various other medical traditions. However, Chinese medicine is also being actively integrated into formal health care systems worldwide.

China and Asia as the forge of global integration

In modern Asia, traditional systems of health care have been incorporated as formal components of national health care since the late 1970s. *China* has had a policy of integrating traditional medicine into national health care for more than six decades, and has an extensive national program in which modern and traditional medicine are combined as formal components of health care provision.

In *India*, the Indian Medicine Central Council Act of 1970 gave an official place in national health programs to the Ayurvedic and Unani medical systems of India (Micozzi 2011). India now has over 200,000 registered traditional medical practitioners, the majority of whom have received their training in government colleges of Ayurvedic or Unani medicine. In both India and China the traditional health sector provides the majority of health care to poor and rural communities which are not considered "profit centers" by the Western biomedical enterprise.

In recent years, other countries have begun to provide increased support for their long-standing traditional medical systems, recognizing that they cannot afford Western medicine.

In *Thailand*, for example, the Ministry of Health promotes the use of 66 traditional medicinal plants in primary health care, based on scientific evidence of their efficacy, as well as on traditional patterns of utilization. The Fourth Public Health Development Plan of Thailand (1977–1981) stated the country's general policy to promote the use of traditional medicinal plants in primary health care. The Seventh Plan (1992–1996) promoted the integration of traditional Thai medicine into community health care and prioritized research on medicinal plants. The Thai Ministry of Public Health also promotes the use of medicinal plants in state-run hospitals and health service centers.

A study by the Royal Tropical Institute of the *Netherlands* found that traditional herbal medicines used in primary health care in Thailand were most effective when self-administered. Since most rural people treat themselves before seeking help from either modern or traditional medical practitioners, herbal medicines offer a low-cost intervention in the early treatment of disease, and provide a safe alternative to the growing problem of self-medication with inappropriate doses and harmful combinations of over-the-counter drugs.

In *Korea*, between 15 and 20 percent of the national health budget is directed to traditional medical services, and government reports indicate that traditional medicine is favored equally by all levels of society. Health insurance coverage is available for oriental medical treatments.

In *Japan*, where physicians have been authorized to prescribe and dispense medications, over two-thirds of all physicians reportedly prescribe herbal medications.

Chapter 18

❀

Chinese Medicine Works

An important correlate of Chinese medicine coming to the West, and spreading globally, is that today it is being subjected to Western biomedical "scientific" testing which has generated convincing scientific "proof." Of course, a critical part of the modern enterprise of medicine in Europe and North America today theoretically involves performing research and regulatory approval on every treatment in practice. While this expectation has the effect of constraining "freedom of choice," it places control of medical practice ultimately in the hands of medical research elites and those who have (pharmaceutical industry) or control (government bureaucracies who collect taxpayers' money) the millions of dollars required to perform acceptable research studies. Western biomedicine has been quick to require the highest standards of research evidence when it comes to alternative therapies like Chinese medicine and acupuncture, for example, but the former U.S. Congressional Office of Technology Assessment (now conveniently abolished) estimated as of the 1990s that 80 percent of medicine as practiced in the U.S. was in fact not based upon acceptable standards of research evidence.

Nonetheless, substantial research efforts have taken place in Asia since the early twentieth century, and during the latter part of that century in North America and Europe as well. Research approaches and standards vary widely and, like medicine itself, are subject to cultural influences. Where the West recognizes the randomized, placebo-controlled, double-blinded clinical trial as the definitive standard for an unambiguous biomedical answer, other societies do not require or encourage their medical communities to secure knowledge in this fashion. In addition, much of the research data that has been gathered is inaccessible in the West due to language differences and difficulty of obtaining publications.

As a result, the scientific communities of China, Japan, Europe, North America, and Australia do not have access to the same information and are not influenced by the same research.

Table 18.1 Research supported by the National Institutes of Health's Office of Alternative Medicine (now the National Center for Complementary and Alternative Medicine)

Medical condition	Therapy
Balance disorders	T'ai chi
Breech presentation birth	Acupuncture and moxibustion
Chronic sinusitis in HIV infection	Traditional Chinese medicine
Common warts	Chinese herbal therapy
Hyperactivity	Acupuncture
Intractable reflex sympathetic dystrophy	*Qi gong*
Menopausal hot flashes	Chinese herbal therapy
Osteoarthritis	Acupuncture
Postoperative oral surgery pain	Acupuncture
Premenstrual syndrome	Traditional Chinese medicine
Unipolar depression	Acupuncture

Problems surrounding research design and methods have come into focus as the Chinese medicine communities of North America and Europe have conducted more research, and as the biomedical community has become better educated about Chinese medicine. In 1991, for example, the U.S. National Institutes of Health created the Office of Alternative Medicine (OAM), which has hosted several conferences dealing with the issue of research study design in the complementary and alternative medicine fields, including Chinese medicine. The OAM has also funded numerous small research grants, many of which have been in the area of Chinese or oriental medicine.

In 1994 the OAM sponsored a workshop in cooperation with the U.S. Food and Drug Administration (FDA). Members of the acupuncture, allopathic medical, and Western scientific communities gave presentations detailing the safety and effectiveness of acupuncture needles. These presentations became the core of a petition that led, in 1996, to the FDA reclassifying acupuncture needles from a Class III or experimental device to a Class II or medical device for use by qualified practitioners with special controls (sterility and single use).

Reclassification of acupuncture needles by the FDA, 1996

During the early 1990s, one of the important aspects of acupuncture under consideration by the U.S. FDA was the safety and effectiveness of acupuncture for asthma. The potent drug bronchodilator inhalers developed for asthma posed severe problems concerning safety of the drugs and the propellants used, which led to many deaths of young people with asthma. Ironically these drugs were originally based on the traditional Chinese herb, *ma huang*, or ephedra, researched by Carl Schmidt at the University of Pennsylvania in the 1930s. Ephedra was later to run into its own safety problems with the FDA, owing to its inappropriate use for weight loss and athletic performance, causing several deaths among young athletes in the early 2000s. This led to a temporary ban and the relegation of associated "over-the-counter" products back behind the pharmacist counter today.

Regarding asthma, the FDA was appropriately concerned with finding other treatments that were effective but also safe. As founding editor of the first medical journal on complementary and alternative medicine, in 1995, the author of this book was impressed by the effectiveness of acupuncture for asthma and other respiratory diseases (challenging the notion that acupuncture was only useful for pain), and had compiled hundreds of references on the use of acupuncture for treating asthma. Meantime, the acupuncture needle had come up at FDA for reclassification from the category of an experimental device (approved for use only in accepted research protocols) to that of a therapeutic device (approved for use in regular clinical practice).

Several dedicated officials at the FDA, including a number of Vietnamese–Americans, obtained permission to work on this approval action in their own time, during evenings and weekends, to speed the approval process. I sent over my hundreds of references on a computer disk, so that the FDA doctors would not need to have their government clerical staff (who are not known for their accuracy, speed, precision or command of the English language) re-enter these technical references. The result was reclassification of acupuncture needles—a victory for science, health and millions of long-suffering Americans.

In 1997 the U.S. National Institutes of Health convened a Consensus Development Conference on acupuncture. For two days, experts in the field presented evidence of the safety and effectiveness of acupuncture in treating specific conditions. The scientific panel that reviewed the presentations noted, in the NIH Consensus Statement of 1997, that while acupuncture was widely practiced and studied in the U.S., much of the research was inconclusive due to problems in design, sample size, and other factors. One particular difficulty involved finding appropriate controls, such as placebos and sham acupuncture groups, since inserting a needle into the skin is not the same as taking a drug or placebo orally. "However," the report concluded:

> promising results have emerged, for example, showing efficacy of acupuncture in adult postoperative and

chemotherapy nausea and vomiting and in postoperative dental pain. There are other situations such as addiction, stroke rehabilitation, headache, menstrual cramps, tennis elbow, fibromyalgia, myofascial pain, osteoarthritis, low back pain, carpal tunnel syndrome, and asthma, in which acupuncture may be useful as an adjunct treatment or an acceptable alternative or be included in a comprehensive management program. Further research is likely to uncover additional areas where acupuncture interventions will be useful. (National Institutes of Health 1997)

Considering that less than two years earlier acupuncture needles had been considered experimental devices in the U.S., this finding marked a significant degree of progress.

In late 1998 the OAM was renamed as the National Center for Complementary and Alternative Medicine and provided with a significant increase in funding. Since its inception this organization has continued to refine and develop its approach to fostering research into complementary therapies, and in the process has involved various established institutions in research projects. Two such institutions—the Center for Addiction and Alternative Medicine Research at the University of Minnesota Medical School and Hennepin County Medical Center, and the Center for Alternative Medicine Pain Research and Evaluation at the University of Maryland School of Medicine—have built their centers around long-term and sustained research efforts in specific areas, which has allowed them to make substantial strides as increased funding became available.

Other national and international organizations, such as the Society for Acupuncture Research (SAR), have emerged out of the broad-based community of acupuncturists, physicians, and researchers interested in the range of research issues posed by this field. SAR holds annual meetings and publishes its proceedings. Among its objectives are scholarly exchange between researchers in the area of acupuncture, as well as other therapies related to Asian medicine; the encouragement of research activities by acupuncturists; and the clarification of research issues such as study design. In 1996 two SAR officers, Richard Hammerschlag (this fortunate author's former mentor during a college research fellowship at City of Hope National Medical Center in Duarte, California) and Stephen Birch, compiled a summary of the most successful and well-designed controlled clinical trials.

Researchers have been successful in obtaining measurable results when exploring such fundamental concepts as *qi*, the channels, acupuncture points, pulse diagnosis, and pattern diagnosis. However, these studies are difficult to design in ways that remain true to the traditional Chinese system, at the same time as obtaining data that will be recognized by the world's scientific community.

For example, Chinese researchers have been pursuing questions about the physiological basis of Chinese medical concepts. One such study examined the nature of kidney yang and reached the conclusion that patients displaying a diagnostic pattern associated with kidney yang vacuity showed low levels of certain steroids (17-hydroxy cortical steroids) in their urine, suggesting a relationship between the concept of kidney yang and the adrenal cortical system.

The study of pulse patterns has been pursued for some time in North America and Europe, as well as China, Japan, and Korea. This research typically includes applying pressure sensors over the radial artery, mimicking the way a clinical practitioner holds his or her fingers during a pulse reading. Pulse patterns are then recorded and correlated to determine the physical foundation of the diagnostic information the practitioner obtains from the pulse. Initial results are intriguing, but too many questions remain about the size and design of the study to make hard data available.

Research concerning channels and acupuncture has relied on a variety of techniques, including the measurement of electrical resistance, thermography, tracing the pathways of injected radioisotopes, and anatomical dissection (although dissection has proved disappointing in this area). Some interesting work is being done to determine how the body's bioelectrical properties transmit information. This approach relates to earlier studies demonstrating that the skin, at many acupuncture points, has a measurably lowered electrical resistance.

Yoshio Manaka, a Japanese surgeon and acupuncturist who did pioneering work in this field during and after World War II, hypothesized the presence of a signaling system he calls "the X-signal system." This concept was drawn from biological theories, texts such as *The Yellow Emperor's Inner Classic*, and observations in his acupuncture clinic. His perspective grew out of exploration of both Chinese and Japanese needling methods, including the gentler needling techniques associated with the school of *meridian therapy* that arose in Japan (Chapter 8).

All of these discussions are preliminary. Even those areas that have generated solid, reproducible results (such as lowered electrical resistance over acupuncture points) raise as many questions as they answer. Scientific research may not prove to be the right vehicle for understanding the fundamental principles of traditional Chinese medicine. It may be that the genius of Chinese medicine in these areas lies in its empirical ability to generalize about the manifestations of incredibly complex biological phenomena in an articulate, internally consistent and clinically useful fashion.

Despite the early and widespread interest in acupuncture, comparatively few studies have been designed in a fashion that renders their results useful to other researchers, clinicians, or policy makers. Rather than focusing on useful observations, many of these "studies" are more in the nature of "de-bunking" experiments worthy of magicians such as the so-called "Amazing Randi"; their agenda is to disprove rather than try to understand this ancient and effective therapy.

Many of the most substantial studies from North American and Europe were presented at the OAM's Workshop on Acupuncture and Consensus Panel of Acupuncture. The clinical work presented was primarily done in five areas: anti-emesis (anti-vomiting) treatment, the management of acute and chronic pain, substance abuse treatment, treatment of paralysis due to stroke, and the treatment of respiratory disease. Good clinical results were also shown in treatment of female infertility, breech presentation, menopause, depression, and urinary dysfunction.

Promise for pain

Pain control is the most widespread application of acupuncture, but it is also one of the most problematic to research. Some of these problems are illustrated by the results of two meta-analyses of studies examining acupuncture in the management of chronic pain. (A meta-analysis is a research method that pools the results of many studies in an effort to reach conclusions more powerful than those generated by an individual study.)

The first meta-analysis combined data from 14 studies that used randomized and controlled trials of acupuncture as a treatment for chronic pain, measuring outcomes in terms of the number of patients whose condition was improved. This study reached a number of conclusions about the relations of study design to research outcomes and determined that acupuncture compares favorably with placebo and conventional treatment.

A second meta-analysis reviewed over 50 studies and compared the quality of published controlled, clinical trials on the basis of research design and specific factors such as randomization, single and double blinding, and numbers of subjects. Investigators determined that the studies favorable to acupuncture were more poorly designed than those that associated negative results with acupuncture. Their conclusion: evidence suggested that the effectiveness of acupuncture as a treatment for chronic pain was doubtful.

A third meta-analysis reviewed the second meta-analysis and found that the authors of the latter had included studies that did not meet appropriate standards and criteria, such as a study that was not controlled and one where laser light was used instead of needles. The authors of this third meta-analysis observed a trend toward improvement of studies over time, suggesting that many poorly designed studies should be viewed as preliminary efforts by investigators who were not sufficiently familiar with acupuncture to design an appropriate study in the first place. This observation points out another problem with research on CAM: many Western scientists who have access to powerful methods and research funding do not have sufficient knowledge of the historic use of CAM remedies to be able to design useful studies. In Germany, by contrast, long known for the high quality of research, the first criterion considered by regulators and scientists is the historic use of CAM treatments.

Putting it all together

These studies highlight some of the key problems in acupuncture research. For example, should the investigator be trained in acupuncture? Is acupuncture appropriate for the condition treated? Does the study allow for adjusting treatment to the individual patient's needs, in accordance with traditional diagnostics? Are outcome measures clear? Will placebo or sham acupuncture be used, and, if so, how will it be administered? Unlike herbal medicine studies, in which a placebo capsule can be administered, subjects in acupuncture studies always know when they've been stuck with a needle, so the concept of "blinding" the participants to the treatment is not valid. Various solutions have been proposed, including comparing acupuncture to other treatments or selecting acupuncture points that are, by traditional standards, irrelevant to the condition being treated. But, so far, no well-accepted study design has emerged from the discussion.

Despite these difficulties, effective studies can be cited. In one study acupuncture patients demonstrated a lower need for postoperative anesthesia following *oral surgery* than a group receiving sham acupuncture treatment, echoing the dramatic experiences of James Reston in President Nixon's diplomatic mission to China in 1971 (see page 185). Another study tracked women with *menstrual pain*; those receiving acupuncture experienced considerably less pain than the placebo and control groups. When *migraine* headache sufferers participated in a controlled trial, acupuncture was significantly effective in controlling the pain. A number of other studies demonstrated the effectiveness of acupuncture for *back pain* and for *osteoarthritis*; one study suggested that the use of acupuncture may produce a considerable cost benefit by *eliminating the need for surgery*.

Research in the area of postoperative *nausea and vomiting* revolves around the use of the acupuncture point which has also been shown to control the nausea of pregnancy and chemotherapy. Other fruitful areas of study include management of *substance addiction*, pulmonary disease, such as *asthma*, and paralysis following *stroke*.

Looking back, as of 1995, there had been approximately 200 randomized controlled trials, 42 review articles, and four meta-analyses performed in the United States alone. The amount of research conducted in *China and Japan* is vast, and translations are becoming more numerous; one English compilation contains 117 Chinese studies on acupuncture and moxibustion. Improvements in study design are occurring in both the East and the West, bringing these two bodies of knowledge closer together.

Like acupuncture research, the field of traditional Chinese medicine in general is plagued with difficulties in designing effective studies. The *cultivation of qi*, such as *qi gong*, is highly personal and does not lend itself to standardized studies. The challenge is to develop an effective control and rule out other variables that might influence the results. However, a number of intriguing investigations have been conducted in China and, more recently, in the United States.

Promising areas of study include the use of *qi gong* for managing *gastritis* and *hypertension*, and for increasing *immune competence*. On the other hand, attempts to study the effects of externally transmitted *qi* have encountered problems with measurement. Some researchers believe *qi* involves measurable portions of the electromagnetic spectrum, while others hypothesize that *qi* exists but cannot be measured by currently available technology, only by its effects on the human body. *Qi* cultivation remains a challenging part of the broad fabric of China's traditional medicine.

Outlook for effective treatments

Forty years ago, few non-Asians had even heard of acupuncture or Chinese medicine. Today, both are well known throughout the West and have become a staple of our cultural vocabulary. Initially opposed by the medical establishment, they have recently gained legal and professional acceptance, which has led to government funding for research at respected academic institutions worldwide. Much about traditional Chinese medicine remains a mystery to Westerners. However, it is clear that this ancient form of health care is moving into the world's medical mainstream. It offers tremendous potential health benefits to those many millions suffering with conditions for which modern Western biomedicine has had little to offer, as well as offering far-reaching possibilities for affordable, effective and sustainable health care that represents true "health care reform."

This most ancient but influential form of medicine has extended beyond the time and space of Greater China to represent a worldwide resource for health and healing in the twenty-first century, using medical practices and technologies that are accessible to everyone, everywhere.

Common Chinese and East Asian Remedies Widely Available and Used in the Western World Today

Several of the most popular herbal remedies used today by millions of people in Europe and North America exist in the Chinese pharmacopeia of *materia medica*. Several of these plant constituents can also be recognized as foods, spices and/or condiments, consistent with Chinese approaches to diet, foods, and herbs as medicine.

Garlic

Throughout history, garlic has been used to flavor food and to treat leprosy, deafness, earaches, flatulence, and scurvy. Today, medical interest focuses primarily on its benefits to the cardiovascular (heart and circulation) system, including lowering cholesterol, blood pressure, and platelet aggregation (clumping of red blood cells that can produce blood clots).

- *Botanical name*: *allium sativum* is the Latin name for what is commonly known as garlic.

- *Part of plant used*: the main bulb plus secondary bulbs known as cloves are used fresh or dried.

- *How it works*: one component, allicin, is believed to act as an antioxidant by stimulating antioxidant enzymes. When allicin breaks down, it produces diallyl disulfide, which has been shown in animal studies to lower cholesterol.

- *Research*: recently, several randomized trials with placebo-control groups have studied garlic's effect on cholesterol. In two meta-analyses, in which numerous studies were correlated and the results evaluated, garlic was shown to decrease cholesterol levels by 9 to 12 percent and to decrease the levels of triglycerides (another fat in the blood) by 8 to 27 percent. In two other investigations, garlic showed no effect on cholesterol or other blood fats. However, these two studies were both small, and some controversy exists regarding the particular garlic supplements used in the research. Additional data suggests that garlic also has some ability to lower blood pressure and reduce blood clots.

- *Uses*: the German Commission E approved garlic for use as an adjunct to diet therapy for the control of cholesterol and other fats in the blood, and as a form of prevention for changes in the blood vessels related to aging. Despite some conflicting data regarding its effectiveness, garlic appears to lower cholesterol and, to a lesser extent, reduce blood pressure.

- *Dosage*: the standard daily dosage is one to four grams of fresh, minced garlic bulb, which may be taken as is, infused in 150 ml of water, pressed to obtain a fluid extract, or combined with alcohol as a tincture. Dried garlic is available in tablets and powder form; dosage is 300 mg, taken two to three times a day.

- *Side effects*: in rare instances, garlic may cause gastrointestinal symptoms such as nausea, vomiting, or diarrhea. Those about to undergo surgery or who are on anti-coagulation medication should not take garlic due to the risk of bleeding. Garlic may reduce blood sugar levels, and therefore should be used with caution by those taking medication to reduce blood glucose. Some find the odor of garlic on the breath and skin unpleasant; this is reduced by taking garlic in tablet or powder form.

- *Interactions*: garlic appears to have blood-thinning properties. Those taking anticoagulant (blood-thinning) medications such as aspirin should refrain from consuming large amounts of garlic, either fresh or commercially processed.

Ginger

Like garlic, ginger is a popular flavoring agent with a long history of medicinal usage. Ancient Sanskrit, Chinese, Greek, Roman, and Arabic texts record its uses for such conditions as stomach ache, diarrhea, and nausea, and today it is included in the national pharmacopeias (official lists of medicines) of Austria, China, Egypt, Germany, Great Britain, Japan, and Switzerland. Contemporary researchers are studying its use for motion sickness, arthritis, and hyperemesis gravidarum (an abnormal condition of pregnancy marked by long-term vomiting, weight loss, and imbalances of fluids and electrolytes).

- *Botanical name*: *zingiber officinalis* is the Latin name; its common name is ginger rhizome.

- *Part of plant used*: the rhizome, the root-like stem that grows underground, is used in remedies and is often (inaccurately) referred to as ginger root.

- *How it works*: ginger's active components include volatile oils that are believed to be beneficial to the heart as well as providing pain relief, sedation, and stimulation to the gastrointestinal tract.

- *Research*: human trials of ginger's effectiveness with motion sickness have had mixed results; some studies support historical claims of effectiveness while others contradict them. One study involved 80 naval cadets exposed to rough sea conditions. Four hours after taking one gram of ginger, the cadets had significantly less vomiting, cold sweating, nausea, and vertigo than those who took a placebo. In another controlled trial, in which individuals were placed in a motorized revolving chair, ginger was found to be more effective for motion sickness than dimenhydrinate, a common motion sickness drug. In yet other studies, ginger was successful in treating *hyperemesis gravidarum*, the nausea and vomiting of pregnancy.

- *Uses*: the German Commission E approved ginger for prevention of motion sickness and relief of dyspepsia (characterized by fullness, heartburn, and other symptoms after eating, possibly due to an underlying condition such as peptic ulcer or gallbladder disease).

- *Dosage*: standard dosage is two to four grams a day of the cut rhizome or dried extract, usually taken in amounts of 250 mg to 1 gram several times a day.

- *Side effects*: there are no known side effects.

- *Interactions*: those taking heart medications, anticoagulant (blood-thinning) medications such as warfarin, or medications used to control blood sugar levels, should check with their physicians before taking ginger to prevent motion sickness, vertigo, migraine, uterine cramps, or arthritis. While no studies have proved that there is an interaction between ginger and these other medications, there is a risk that ginger can either block or increase the effects of some of these medications.

Gingko

The world's oldest surviving tree, gingko has been used for medicinal purposes since ancient times. More than 400 scientific studies have been conducted in the past 30 years, many of them by W. Schwabe Co. of Germany, which produces the extract known as EGb 761. Unlike many herbs, such as garlic and ginger, which can be used in their natural state, gingko leaves and leaf extracts are not reliable methods for achieving the desired results, and a standardized dose in the form of EGb 761 is now recommended.

Historically, gingko was used to treat asthma and chilblains (swelling of the hands and feet due to exposure to damp cold). Today, research concentrates on studying the effects of EGb 761 on the blood supply to the brain, and how enhancing that blood supply may help in organic mental disorders (primarily dementia), arterial disease, vertigo, and tinnitus.

- *Botanical name*: *gingko biloba* is the Latin name; common names include duck foot tree, maidenhair tree, and silver apricot.

- *Part of plant used*: leaf extract is prepared according to a proprietary process and marketed as EGb 761.

- *How it works*: two groups of active constituents—terpene lactones and carbohydrates known as gingko flavone glycocides—are thought to improve circulation by dilating the arteries and capillaries, and inhibiting platelet aggregation in the blood. They also have antioxidant properties, which require the synergistic action of other substances found in the plant.

- *Research*: many studies have demonstrated the positive effects of gingko on the blood supply to the brain. In a large 1997 study published in the *Journal of the American Medical Association*, the effects of EGb 761 on dementia were studied in a one-year, randomized, double-blind, placebo-controlled trial. A group of 202 patients with mild to moderate dementia caused by Alzheimer's disease or loss of blood to the brain were shown to improve reasoning, learning, judgment, social functioning, and daily living skills when given gingko. A 1999 study, comparing gingko extracts to the common dementia drugs known as cholinesterase inhibitors, showed that gingko was equally effective as the drug in delaying or moderating symptoms of dementia. Research in the Himalayas involved 44 men who had previously experienced altitude sickness. In eight days, they ascended to a base camp at 14,700 feet, with periodic ascents to even higher elevations. Those taking gingko experienced none of the headache, nausea, dizziness, and other symptoms normally caused by such high altitude. Another 1999 report suggests that gingko may be an effective treatment for tinnitus (ringing in the ear). A new and novel area of study is the use of gingko for improving sexual function in those taking SSRI (selective serotonin reuptake inhibitors) anti-depressants. A geriatric patient seeking memory enhancement discovered this side benefit, prompting a study of 63 people. More effective for women (who showed 91 percent improvement) than for men (76 percent improvement), gingko reportedly had a positive effect on all four phases of the response cycle: desire, excitement, orgasm, and afterglow. The mechanism of this effect is not yet fully understood, and additional research is needed before such use can be generally recommended.

- *Uses*: the German Commission E approved gingko for symptomatic treatment of disturbed mental performance found in organic brain syndrome, including degenerative dementia and dementia caused by loss of blood to the brain. It was also approved in Germany for use in blocked arteries and for vertigo and tinnitus.

- *Dosage*: a standard daily dosage is 120 mg of EGb 761, divided into two or three doses.

- *Side effects*: gingko rarely causes any side effects. Occasionally some people experience dizziness, headache, stomach upset and/or heart palpitations.

- *Interactions*: gingko has blood-thinning properties and should not be used while taking anticoagulant (blood-thinning) medications such as aspirin or warfarin. Use with non-steroidal anti-inflammatory drugs should be avoided until safety research is more conclusive.

Ginseng

For more than 5000 years, the Chinese have viewed ginseng as the most powerful and versatile remedy in their extensive herbal pharmacy. Its genus name, *Panax*, has the same Greek root as the word "panacea," which means "cure all." The common name *gin* (man) *seng* (essence) is derived from the Chinese ideogram meaning "crystallization of the essence of the earth in the form of a man." The therapeutic use of ginseng is described in *The Divine Husbandman's Classic of the Materia Medica* (*Shen Nong Ben Cao Jing*), the classic work attributed to Shen Nong (see pages 14–15), the Divine Husbandman and Fire Emperor (2737–2697 BCE), although it was not actually written until 220 CE (see Part I, especially Chapter 6, for further detail). In Chinese and other Asian medical traditions, dried ginseng is used as a tonic to stimulate and balance *qi*, the vital energy of the body and mind. Today, ginseng is being studied for its effects on a wide variety of conditions, including mental and physical stress and fatigue, sexual performance, and age-related complaints.

- *Botanical name*: there are several species of ginseng, including American ginseng (*Panax quinquefolius*), Korean or Chinese ginseng (*Panax ginseng*), and Siberian ginseng (*Eleutherococcus senticosus*). All are used medicinally and possess different qualities. The German Commission E and the discussion below focus exclusively on Korean or Chinese ginseng (*Panax ginseng*). (See also page 60.)

- *Part of plant used*: the root of this slow-growing perennial is used medicinally.

- *How it works*: the most important active constituents of ginseng are thought to be the carbohydrates known as ginsenosides. They are part of the process by which ginseng has an indirect effect on the pituitary gland, increasing the production of adrenal steroids. This promotes a general increase in resistance to the harmful effects of biological, chemical, or physical stress. Ginseng is also thought to increase the nerve impulses that stimulate muscles, modify brain waves, and balance the brain–hormone interface, which would account for this herb's ability to offset the effects of fatigue. Ginseng lowers blood sugar and promotes the release of nitric oxide, which creates an antioxidant effect and improves circulation by dilating the veins.

- *Research*: several investigations, one of which was a three-month, randomized, placebo-controlled trial, showed that users of ginseng had a significant increase in scores on tests measuring quality of life. Volunteers in another study demonstrated improved speed and accuracy when performing mathematical calculations after taking ginseng. Other research subjects have demonstrated reduced fatigue and increased performance while taking the herb. Thirty patients undergoing heart bypass surgery recovered more quickly with less swelling on ginseng, and a study of 36 newly diagnosed diabetes patients showed improvements on ginseng in a double-blind, placebo-controlled study. Unfortunately, many of the other studies involving ginseng were poorly designed and executed, and so cannot be considered conclusive.

- *Uses*: the German Commission E approved ginseng as a tonic to strengthen and invigorate those with fatigue, debility, and declining concentration.

- *Dosage*: the standard daily dosage is one to two grams of root or the equivalent; preparations should be standardized to include 10 mg of ginsenosides.

- *Side effects*: it is rare for side effects to be encountered. Occasionally people experience headaches, insomnia, anxiety, skin rashes, and increases in blood pressure. Ginseng may alter estrogen levels, causing vaginal bleeding and other symptoms, and theoretically could affect hormonally driven tumors. Because it lowers blood sugar, those who have low blood sugar to begin with may want to use extra caution. Ginseng's stimulant effect may make it inadvisable for those with bipolar disease.

- *Interactions*: there have been reports of a possible interaction between Chinese or Korean ginseng and the blood thinner warfarin, that may result in decreased effectiveness of the blood-thinning medication. Those taking warfarin, or any non-steroidal anti-inflammatory drug, should refrain from taking Chinese or Korean ginseng.

Southeast Asian
Herbal Remedies

Appendix II lists herbs from the "Spice Islands" of Southeast Asia with their medicinal properties, that are commonly available today in the West. The plant chemicals present in herbs and spices protect the plant from the oxidizing effects of the sun, from microbes, and from insect and animal predators, as well as allowing them to compete with other plants for soil, water, and nutrients. The biologically active plant chemicals in turn have properties as anti-oxidants, antibiotics, and other medicinal activities. These properties made spices invaluable for preserving meats and foods, making them precious to Europeans in the era before refrigeration or canning of foods, thanks to many of the same properties that make them safe and effective herbal remedies today.

Allium sativum (garlic)

Garlic has long been used in Southeast Asia as a medicinal food. In modern herbal medicine, it was initially used as an *anti-infective* agent and subsequently became popular for its antihypertensive and *lipid-lowering* effects. In the U.S., sales of garlic products have soared in recent years, generating over $60 million in the year 2000. Garlic has lipid-lowering, anti-thrombotic, antihypertensive, antioxidant and immunomodulatory properties.

Several trials have shown the effectiveness of garlic in reducing total and low-density lipoprotein (LDL)-cholesterol. Garlic's reported anti-platelet, fibrinolytic and anti-atherosclerotic effects in some studies need to be better defined and understood in terms of their benefits in various neurological and cerebrovascular conditions. In a recent analysis performed by the Agency for Healthcare Research and Quality (AHRQ), it was concluded that garlic may have short-term, positive lipid-lowering and encouraging anti-thrombotic effects. All these effects can be expected to *reduce the risk of cardiovascular diseases and heart attack and stroke.*

Boswellia serrata (frankincense)

Boswellia is a commonly used ingredient in herbal preparations. It comes from a gum tree that grows in South and Southeast Asia. In Christian belief it was one of the traditional gifts brought from the East by the Three Magi at Epiphany. Its effects are similar to those of corticosteroid anti-inflammatory drugs, but without the side effects. Boswellic acids are reported to have significant analgesic, anti-inflammatory and complement-inhibitory properties. In one study involving 30 patients with *osteoarthritis* of the knee, those who received *Boswellia* tree extract reported a significant improvement in their knee pain, range of motion, and walking distance. In another study of *rheumatoid arthritis* patients, a special gum extract of *Boswellia serrata* resulted in a significant improvement of symptoms of pain and swelling. These results are promising.

Capsicum annuum (chilli pepper)

Common names of this plant/herb include cayenne pepper, paprika, red pepper, bird pepper and Peruvian pepper. The preparations of this plant are used in topical creams and ointments. It is commonly used for pain related to *herpes zoster* and *diabetic neuropathy.* Many use it for *osteoarthritic* pain. Some basic science studies have shown that it reduces pain by depleting Substance P, a chemical pain transmitter. There are also reports of the herb desensitizing neurons.

Curcuma longa (turmeric)

The active ingredient, *curcumin*, of this commonly-used spice in Southeast Asian curry dishes has *anti-inflammatory* and *lipid-lowering* effects. It is one of the three components of traditional curry spices, together with *coriander* and *cumin*, and sometimes *chilli pepper* (see above). Curcumin's lipid-lowering effects observed in animal experiments are attributed to changes in fatty acid metabolism and facilitating the conversion of cholesterol to bile acids. There are also reports of its benefit in patients with *osteoarthritis*. The benefits of turmeric are not conclusively proven, but its use as a spice in an overall healthy diet is prudent.

Withania somnifera (winter cherry)

Basic science studies suggest that this herb may have anti-inflammatory, antioxidant, immunomodulatory and hemopoietic, as well as *anti-aging* properties. It may also have a positive influence on the endocrine and central nervous systems. The mechanisms of these proposed actions require additional clarification. Several observational and randomized studies have reported its usefulness in the treatment of *arthritic* conditions.

Zingiber officinalis (ginger)

Ginger is widely used in Southeast Asia, most commonly for control of *nausea* and *osteoarthritic* pain. Several studies have shown its benefit in controlling nausea associated with pregnancy, motion sickness and anesthesia, and some studies have demonstrated its usefulness in the treatment of osteoarthritis.

Memory, cognitive improvement, and anti-aging

Many of these plants and their products have been reported to have anti-aging effects. Examples of these effects include *improvements in memory and cognition*. Based on the available scientific information, these herbs or their extracts have not been found to be of proven value. Additional studies are required to validate their reported benefits.

Table II.I Southeast Asian herbal remedies

Genus, species (common English name)	Conditions and results
Allium sativum (garlic)	*Hyperlipidemia*: results in improved levels of lipids (lipid lowering, anti-thrombotic, anti-hypertensive, immunomodulatory)
Boswellia serrata (frankincense)	*Arthritis*: some reports of beneficial effects (anti-inflammatory)
Capsicum annuum (chilli pepper, paprika)	*Cluster headaches, neuropathy and arthritis*: improvement reported in some studies *External*: rubifacient, blocks pain neurotransmitter-substance P, depletes substance P, desensitizes the sensory neurons *Internal*: reduces platelet aggregation and triglycerides, and improves blood flow
Curcuma longa (turmeric)	*Functional gall bladder problems*: increase in secretin and bicarbonate output *Hyperlipidemia*: some studies report improvement in cholesterol levels (fatty acid metabolism alteration and decrease in serum lipid peroxide levels) *Osteoarthritis*: some studies report positive results (anti-inflammatory)
Commiphora guggulu (guggul lipid)	*Hyperlipidemia*: improved lipid levels noted (antagonist of farnesoid X receptors)
Withania somnifera (winter cherry)	*Arthritis*: some studies report improvement (anti-inflammatory)
Zingiber officinalis (ginger)	Anti-emetic (carminative, local effect on stomach) Reduces nausea *Osteoarthritis*: some studies report benefit (anti-inflammatory—inhibits cyclo-oxygenase pathways, prostaglandin PGE2) and leukotriene (LTB4) synthesis

Biographies

Marc Micozzi, MD, PhD is the Founder and Director of the Policy Institute for Integrative Medicine at Thomas Jefferson University Hospital. He is a former Executive Director of the College of Physicians and Director of the National Museum of Health and Medicine. For many years, Dr. Micozzi has pioneered vital health information to professionals and consumers, collaborating with former U.S. Surgeon General C. Everett Koop and other leaders in the growing wellness movement. In the early 1990s, he frequently shared the speaker's podium and the radio and television airwaves with leaders such as Drs. Andrew Weil, Deepak Chopra, Mehmet Oz, and Dean Ornish. Dr. Micozzi lives in Bethesda, Maryland, and Rockport, Massachusetts.

Kevin Ergil, MA, MS, LAc, Diplomate in Oriental Medicine (NCCAOM), FNAAOM, FAAPM is a Professor at the Finger Lakes School of Acupuncture and Oriental Medicine of NYCC. He is a practitioner of traditional Chinese medicine and a medical anthropologist. He has served as a director of the Society for Acupuncture Research and as a member of the advisory board. He is a past president of the American College of Traditional Chinese Medicine, San Francisco, CA, and was the founding Dean of the Pacific College of Oriental Medicine, New York Campus. He was Director of Research and Chair of the Department of Acupuncture at the New York College for Wholistic Health Education & Research (now the New York College for Health Professions).

Laurel S. Gabler, BA, MSc, originally from Amagansett, New York, is a Rhodes Scholar currently reading for a PhD in Public Health at the University of Oxford. She graduated from Stanford University in 2006 with honors in Psychology and earned her MSc with distinction in Global Health Science from Oxford in 2009. Her undergraduate honors research focused on patient-provider interactions and prognosis of neuro-critical care patients in the Stanford ICU. Since graduation Laurel has worked and conducted research in both the developed and developing world on projects ranging from the genetics of recurrent early-onset depression to the efficacy of acupuncture in the U.S. to HIV/AIDS awareness in East Africa to traditional medicine in Thailand (while she was on a Luce Scholarship). Laurel's current research focuses on the health-seeking behaviours and health system utilization of people in rural Makwanpur, Nepal, a project for which she received a Fulbright research grant. Laurel plans to start medical school in 2012, upon completion of her PhD. It is her ultimate intention to work as a public health practitioner, educator and clinician in the developing world—to do her part to reverse the brain drain that draws health professionals from the developing to the developed world.

Kerry Palanjian, MBA earned both his BA and MBA degrees from The Pennsylvania State University. In 1994, seeing the growing need for an effective stress reduction tool that would fit easily within the existing corporate structure in the U.S., Kerry completed three levels of certification in Shiatsu at The Pennsylvania School of Shiatsu and created Shiatsu On-Site. The same year, he received National Certification in Therapeutic Massage and Bodywork. Kerry has also served as an instructor in the Advanced Studies Program at the Connecticut Center for Massage. He has also received awards for both excellence in management, and distinguished customer service in the natural foods industry, where he has additionally worked for over 25 years. He continues to work at Essene Natural Foods in Philadelphia, PA, a store that has received numerous Best of PhillyTM awards since its inception in 1969. He continues to practice, teach, and lecture throughout the U.S., including guest-lecturing at a major university's college of nursing, as well as Gloucester County College and Montgomery County Community College.

References

AOBTA (2001) "General definition and scope of practice." Voorhees, NJ: American Organization of Body Therapies of Asia.

Brun, V. (2003) "Traditional Thai Medicine." In Selin, H. and Shapiro, H. (eds.) *Medicine Across Cultures: History and Practice of Medicine in Non-Western Cultures*. Boston and London: Kluwer Academic Publishers.

Chokevivat, Vichai *et al.* (2005) "The Use of Traditional Medicine in the Thai Health Care System." World Health Organization Regional Office for South East Asia: Regional Consultation on Development of Traditional Medicine in the South East Asia Region, Pyongyang, DPR Korea, 22–24 June. Document no. 9.

Chokevivat, V. and Chuthaputti, A. (2005) "The Role of Thai Traditional Medicine in Health Promotion." Bangkok: Ministry of Public Health, Department for the Development of Thai Traditional and Alternative Medicine.

Chuakul, W. *et al.* (1997) *Medicinal Plants in Thailand, Volume 2*. Bangkok: Mahidol University, Department of Pharmaceutical Botany.

Cowmeadow, O. (1992) *The Art of Shiatsu*. Rockport, MA: Element Books.

Fabrega Jr, H. (1997) *Evolution of Healing and Sickness*. Berkeley: University of California.

Hirayama, T. (1982) (1981 on p.136) "Relationship of soybean paste soup to gastric cancer." *Nutrition and Cancer 3*, 223–33.

Hsu, E. (1989) "Outline of the history of Chinese medicine in Europe." *Journal of Chinese Medicine 29*, 1, 28–32.

Kushi, M. and Jack, A. (1983) *The Cancer Prevention Diet: Michio Kushi's Nutritional Blueprint for the Relief and Prevention of Disease*. New York: St. Martin's Press.

Masunaga, S. and Oshashi, W. (1977) *Zen Shiatsu*. New York, NY: Japan Publications.

Micozzi, M.S. (1983) "Traditional Ethnomedicines: Four Levels of Effect?" Washington, DC: Human Organization, Society for Applied Anthropology.

Micozzi, M.S. (2007) *Complementary and Integrative Medicine in Cancer Control and Prevention*. New York: Springer.

Micozzi, M.S. (2011) *Vital Healing: Energy, Mind and Spirit in Traditional Medicines of India, Tibet and the Middle East – Middle Asia*. London and Philadelphia: Singing Dragon.

National Institutes of Health (1997) "Acupuncture." *NIH Consensus Statement 15*, 5, 1–34.

Oleson, T. (1996) *Auriculotherapy Manual*. Los Angeles, CA: Health Care Alternatives.

Said, E. (1978) *Orientalism*. New York: New World Books.

Saito, K. (2001) *This is the Shiatsu from Japan*. Vancouver: Japanese Shiatsu Association of Canada.

Salguero, P. C. (2003) *A Thai Herbal: Traditional Recipes for Health and Harmony*. Chiang Mai: Silkworm Books.

Salguero, P. C. (2006) *The Spiritual Healings of Traditional Thailand*. Scotland: Findhorn Press.

Sattilaro, A. (1982) *Recalled by Life*. New York: Avon Books.

Sergel, D. (1989) *The Macrobiotic Way of Zen Shiatsu*. New York, NY: Japan Publications.

Teas, J. *et al.* (1984) "Dietary seaweed (laminaria) and mammary carcinogenesis in rats." *Cancer Research*, 44, 2758–61.

Tillyard, E.M.W. (1959) *The Elizabethan World Picture*. London: Vintage.

Wittfogel, Karl A. (1957) *Oriental Despotism: A Comparative Study of Total Power*. New Haven and London: Yale University Press.

Yamamoto, S. and McCarty, P. (1993) *Whole Health Shiatsu*. New York, NY: Japan Publications.

Further Reading

Chang, K.C. (1977) *Food in Chinese Culture: Anthropological and Historical Perspectives*. New Haven and London: Yale University Press.

Chomchalow, N., Bansiddhi, J. and MacBaine, C. (2003) *Amazing Thai Medicinal Plants*. Bangkok: Horticultural Research Institute Department of Agriculture.

Huang Di Nei Jing Su Wen (1979) "Simple Questions." *The Yellow Emperor's Inner Classic (Classic of Internal Medicine)*. Beijing: People's Health Publishing House.

Huang Di Nei Jing Su Wen (1979) "Spiritual Pivot." *The Yellow Emperor's Inner Classic (Classic of Internal Medicine)*. Beijing: People's Health Publishing House.

Mullholland, J. (1989) *Herbal Medicine in Paediatrics: Translation of a Thai Book of Genesis*. Canberra: Australian National University.

Mullholland, J. (1997a) "Thai traditional medicine: ancient thought and practice in a Thai context." *Journal of the Siam Society,* 67, 2, 80–115.

Mullholland, J. (1997b) "Traditional Thai medicine in Thailand." *Hemisphere 23*, 4, 224–229.

Newbold, V. (1988) "Macrobiotics: An Approach to the Achievement of Health, Happiness and Harmony." In Esko, E. (ed.) *Doctors Look at Macrobiotics*. New York: Japan Publications.

Salguero, P. C. (2004) *Encyclopedia of Thai Massage: A Complete Guide to Traditional Thai Massage Therapy and Acupressure*. Scotland: Findhorn Press.

Salguero, Pierce C. (2007) *Traditional Thai Medicine: Buddhism, Animism, Ayurveda*. Prescott: Hohm Press.

Saralamp, P. *et al.* (1996) *Medicinal Plants in Thailand. Volume 1*. Bangkok: Department of Pharmaceutical Botany, Mahidol University.

Subcharoen, S. (1989) *Thai Traditional Medicine: System and Practice*. Faculty of Graduate Studies, Mahidol University.

Index